CATEGORY - PT. CE,

Patient-Centered Ca

Series Editors

Moira Stewart,
Judith Belle Brown
and
Thomas R Freeman

```
DRS BRAY, SMITH, PATEL
TANNA & WHITER
St. Andrews Medical Practice
50 Oakleigh Road North
Whetstone London N20 9EX
Tel: 020 8445 0475
```

Chronic Fatigue Syndrome

A patient-centered approach

Campbell Murdoch
and
Harriet Denz-Penhey

Radcliffe Medical Press

Radcliffe Medical Press Ltd
18 Marcham Road
Abingdon
Oxon OX14 1AA
United Kingdom

www.radcliffe-oxford.com
The Radcliffe Medical Press electronic catalogue and online ordering facility. Direct sales to anywhere in the world.

© 2002 The authors

All rights reserved. No part of this publication may be reproduced, stored in a retrieval system or transmitted, in any form or by any means, electronic, mechanical, photocopying, recording or otherwise without the prior permission of the copyright owner.

British Library Cataloguing in Publication Data

A catalogue record for this book is available from The British Library.

ISBN 1 85775 907 9

Typeset by Aarontype Ltd, Easton, Bristol
Printed and bound by TJ International Ltd, Padstow, Cornwall

Contents

Series editors' introduction	vii
About the authors	ix
Acknowledgments	xi
Introduction *Campbell Murdoch and Harriet Denz-Penhey*	xiii
1 The magnitude of the problem of chronic fatigue syndrome	1
2 The illness experience	27
3 Is there a disease called chronic fatigue syndrome?	47
4 Understanding the whole person	77
5 Mad, bad or dangerous to know? The societal context of chronic fatigue syndrome	99
6 The patient–clinician relationship	115
7 Finding the appropriate treatment for chronic fatigue syndrome	137
Index	163

Series editors' introduction

The strength of medicine in curing many infectious diseases and some of the chronic diseases has also led to a key weakness. Some believe that medicine has abdicated its caring role and, in doing so, has not only alienated the public to some extent, but also failed to uphold its promise to 'do no harm'. One hears many stories of patients who have been technically cured but feel ill or who feel ill but for whom no satisfactory diagnosis is possible. In focusing so much attention on the nature of the disease, medicine has neglected the person who suffers the disease. Redressing this 20th century phenomenon required a new definition of medicine's role for the 21st century. A new clinical method, which has been developed during the 1980s and 1990s, has attempted to correct the flaw, to regain the balance between curing and caring. It is called a Patient-Centered Clinical Method and has been described and illustrated in *Patient-Centered Medicine: Transforming the Clinical Method* (Stewart et al., 1995) of which the 2nd edition is being prepared for publication in early 2003. In the 1995 book, conceptual, educational and research issues were elucidated in detail. The patient-centered conceptual framework from that book is used as the structure for each book in the series introduced here; it consists of six interactive components to be considered in every patient–practitioner interaction.

The first component is to assess the two modes of ill health; disease and illness. In addition to assessing the disease process, the clinician explores the patient's illness experience. Specifically, the practitioner considers how the patient feels about being ill, what the patient's ideas are about the illness, what impact the illness is having on the patient's functioning and what he or she expects from the clinician.

The second component is an integration of the concepts of disease and illness with an understanding of the whole person. This includes an awareness of the patient's position in the lifecycle and the social context in which they live.

The third component of the method is the mutual task of finding common ground between the patient and the practitioner. This consists of three key areas: mutually defining the problem, mutually defining the goals of management/treatment, and mutually exploring the roles to be assumed by the patient and the practitioner.

The fourth component is to use each visit as an opportunity for prevention and health promotion. The fifth component takes into consideration that each encounter with the patient should be used to develop the helping relationship;

the trust and respect that evolves in the relationship will have an impact on other components of the method. The sixth component requires that, throughout the process, the practitioner is realistic in terms of time, availability of resources and the amount of emotional and physical energy needed.

However, there is a gap between the description of the clinical method and its application in practice. The series of books presented here attempts to bridge that gap. Written by international leaders in their field, the series represents clinical explications of the patient-centered clinical method. Each volume deals with a common and challenging problem faced by practitioners. In each book, current thinking is organized in a similar way, reinforcing and illustrating the patient-centered clinical method. The common format begins with a description of the burden of illness, followed by chapters on the illness experience, the disease, the whole person, the patient–practitioner relationship and finding common ground, including current therapeutics.

The book series is international, to date representing Norway, Canada, Australia, New Zealand and the USA. This is a testament to the universality of the values and concepts inherent in the patient-centered clinical method. The work of not only the authors, but others who have studied patients, has reinforced a virtually identical series of six components (Little *et al.*, 2001; Stewart, 2001). We feel that there is an emerging international definition of patient-centered practice which is represented in this book series.

The vigor of any clinical method is proven in the extent to which it is applicable in the clinical setting. It is anticipated that this series will inform further development of the clinical method and move thinking forward in this important aspect of medicine.

Moira Stewart PhD
Judith Belle Brown PhD
Thomas R Freeman MD, CCFP

References

Little P, Everitt H, Williamson I *et al.* (2001) Preferences of patients for patient-centred approach to consultation in primary care: observational study. *BMJ.* **322**(7284): 468–72.

Stewart M (2001) Towards a global definition of patient-centred care. *BMJ.* **322**(7284): 444–5.

Stewart M, Brown JB, Weston WW *et al.* (1995) *Patient-Centered Medicine: transforming the clinical method.* Sage Publications Inc, Thousand Oaks, CA.

About the authors

Campbell Murdoch MB, ChB, MD, PhD, FRCGP, FRNZCGP is a Family Physician in rural practice in Winton, Southland, New Zealand and is also Editor of the *New Zealand Family Physician*. He was Professor and Chair of the Department of General Practice, Dunedin School of Medicine from 1983 to 1992, and a pioneer in research and clinical management of chronic fatigue syndrome at a time when the syndrome had a high prevalence in New Zealand. From 2002, he will be Professor and Head, Rural Clinical School, University of Western Australia, Kalgoorlie, WA.

Harriet Denz-Penhey B Theol, PhD is currently working in medical education in West Australia.

She has a strong research interest in patient self-care in serious illness, with particular concern as to what patients can do to improve their quality of life in addition to what medicine can do to help. Her PhD was a study of patients with a poor prognosis (less than 10% chance of survival) but who had quality outcomes. She recognises the need to support general practitioners in developing patient-centered clinical care in the practice setting.

Acknowledgments

We thank the very many patients who have contributed to our knowledge of this illness. We thank them for being so open with the stories of their lives.

Special thanks to Annie and Bruce for their support and encouragement as we wrote, edited and re-edited this book.

Introduction

This volume is part of a series of books on Patient-Centered Care. It is different from most other books in the series because it is about an illness which has not yet qualified as a disease. There is, therefore, no objective proof, as would be found in the case of breast cancer or diabetes mellitus, which assists the physician to make a diagnosis or a prognosis. People have developed alarming and multiple symptoms and their doctors and the research community have searched long and hard for explanations. However, so far, all we can do is to describe the illness in such terms as *chronic fatigue syndrome, chronic immunodeficiency and fatigue syndrome, myalgic encephalomyelitis syndrome,* or *fibromyalgia syndrome.* For the modern doctor, this is a difficult if not intolerable situation to be in, and the discomfort intrudes upon our consultations with these patients. To protect ourselves we call these people 'heartsink' patients, choosing to blame the victim rather than admit diagnostic defeat.

The people who have the symptoms are in an even worse predicament because not only do they have symptoms which have shattered their whole lives, they also have to endure the indignity of not being believed or they have to spend a lot of energy finding a doctor who does believe in them and their symptoms. Everyone finds it very difficult to suffer from something which does not exist and they have tended to go from doctor to doctor for a name if not a diagnosis or to join support groups whose purpose seems to be not only mutual support but also action to force the medical profession and researchers into authenticating the symptoms through a proven diagnosis.

The lesson of chronic fatigue syndrome (CFS) seems to be that having an accepted disease is so far an essential ticket of entry to the modern patient–doctor relationship, that simply being a person is not enough. There is no greater evidence of the prevalence of a doctor and disease-centered approach than that people are only accepted as patients if the tests are positive. In this book we address the central concern of the patient and their illness experience in addition to the very real necessity of addressing the biomedical issues of care. These people may be ill with CFS, and the symptoms require attention, but they may also suffer from any of the multitude of other medical conditions that can afflict humankind and too often symptoms of other conditions are disregarded.

We believe that the doctor and disease-centered culture which surrounds modern medicine is a major reason for the discomfort and suffering experienced by persons with CFS. We understand their frustration with the prejudices which they face but do not believe that the answer lies in necessarily proving a physical or organic cause for the problem. The jury is still out on whether viral, immunological, endocrine or psychological causes are predominant in its causation. What is definite is that each sufferer is a person who has been diminished and disabled by their symptoms. The patient-centered approach recognises the suffering and the illness experience, and is sufficient to gain access to the doctor. Together, doctor and patient can work to alleviate the difficulties and work towards an improved quality of life.

The history of CFS has been a war zone where those who hold firm views on causation have fought to gain the advantage. Here we seek a peace process armed with the facts about a difficult problem. We hope our approach will be helpful to all those who have to live with CFS either professionally or personally.

Campbell Murdoch
Harriet Denz-Penhey
June 2002

The magnitude of the problem of Chronic Fatigue Syndrome

Case study

Wendy Jones, aged 25, is married to Willie, a self-employed plumber who has recently been retrenched from his Hospital Board position and is attempting to start himself in business with his redundancy payments. They have two children, Jack who is nearly three years old and Samantha, aged 10 months. Wendy had always been in good health and appeared to be coping well for the first two months after the birth. Then she stopped breast feeding six months ago and almost immediately developed the worst flu of her life. Since then she has had a nightmare illness with recurring muscle pains, severe headaches, lack of sleep, memory loss and lack of sexual desire. She is so sick that she now feels unable to look after the baby and toddler. She has attended her family doctor, Dr Alan Rose, on what seem innumerable occasions, but, in spite of numerous blood tests and investigations, she has been given no explanation for her symptoms.

Her father is a successful accountant and he and his wife have always felt unhappy about her choice of husband. They have heard of chronic fatigue syndrome (CFS) from friends in the US and want to send Wendy to a clinic in Los Angeles for more tests. Willie refuses to let her go, remembering that his father-in-law refused to help him financially with his business, and feels that his in-laws are exaggerating the whole problem just to come between them. Wendy is very tearful when she consults her doctor and she reports that Willie has been working late and coming home smelling of alcohol.

Evaluating the drama not the symptoms

While the scenario which is described here is not all that common, most family doctors and indeed most families have had the experience of being in a situation where the ground has seemed to move around them. Consultations in medicine have been classified as being of three types; routines, rituals and dramas (Marinker, 1983), and there is definitely a drama unfolding here. A drama has been defined as an encounter involving uncertainty, conflict, emotion, lack of common ground, family discord or diagnosis of an illness with grave implications. The symptoms of tiredness, weariness, fatigue or lack of energy are very common symptoms in primary medical care; indeed, fatigue is the seventh most common presenting complaint in general practice (McWhinney, 1997). This is a problem in itself, because everyone has experienced the feeling of tiredness and we all tend to interpret it in our own light.

However, there is a paradox here which few doctors seem to understand, and it is that the illness of CFS has little to do with the symptom of fatigue. Fatigue on its own is a rather benign feeling that follows exertion and precedes sleep. CFS is a drama full of symptoms where the fatigue comes for no reason and sleep seems either to be elusive or unrefreshing. Perhaps this is the reason why it has taken 60 years for this syndrome to become recognized and classified. The problem is that many doctors, like Wendy's doctor, concentrate on the individual symptoms such as fatigue, rather than taking in the *big picture*.

> Picture the scene. Here is a potentially idyllic picture of a modern nuclear family, two partners, deeply in love, with two small children. Then it all falls apart, a fact which is obvious to Wendy, her husband Willie, their respective parents, and even little Jack could tell you that *Mama isn't what she used to be.* The man in the corner shop knows that Wendy has a big problem and all her friends at the kindergarten have noticed that she does not come to the committee meetings any more. As in all drama, there has been a change that is vivid, tense and striking. Wendy is the central character; she has changed and the supporting cast of her partner, her children, her parents, her in-laws and her doctor are all changed as a result.

Testimony: starting with the persons

Evidence-based medicine is now given great emphasis in medical journals but one of the weaknesses of the movement is its limited view of what constitutes evidence. The meaning often approximates to what can be scientifically proven but, in real life, evidence is all about the testimony of witnesses under oath. Harvey Cox (1973) related this kind of evidence to his boyhood memories of members of his church testifying to their faith and has emphasized the importance of allowing the evidence of human experience to be heard.

> The idea of testimony itself remains powerful and essential: to try to give voice to what is so patently interior, to stammer at its unspeakableness, to

try so hard to be honest to your inner reality, to know when it is over, that you have failed but that the failure itself was necessary.

If Wendy had been allowed to testify to what had happened to her in these few months she would have found it difficult to tell the story without emotion. If a journalist, or a dramatist, had gone to the Jones household in the middle of all this, there would have been a front-page story or a play to be produced, but Dr Rose is strangely unmoved by the situation. He is so conditioned to looking for what has been described before and evaluated by others that he refuses to recognize new problems or even variations on a theme. He would feel very uncomfortable when confronted by the emotional account of the falling apart of the individual and her family. He would call it subjective, even purely subjective, and would want to cool things down and make it objective. He wants to exclude the life experience of his patients from his thinking. Unless he can find their symptoms under a heading on the pages of a textbook and relate them to physical findings on examination, or specific diagnostic findings on investigation, he is not prepared to say anything about what is wrong, and he remains silent as things fall more and more apart.

This is a book about the person-centered approach to CFS and so it is appropriate that it should start with a bias towards persons. One of the persons who is writing is JCM and, unlike most writers of academic texts, he writes as a person, but he feels guilty about the personal pronouns.

'Before 1983, I had never seen anything that looked remotely like the drama of CFS in any of my patients. From 1968–77 I had been in full-time general practice, and thereafter in an academic practice. Sometimes I felt that perhaps I had missed some insight back then and so I re-examined notes from approximately 5000 consultations carried out in full time practice in 1975. There were always dramas: the 35-year-old woman who had a normal baby and who 10 days later took her own life by swallowing the capsules which her doctor had given her for sleeping; the 31-year-old who died of systemic lupus erythematosis (SLE); the 44-year-old lady with acute leukaemia. The young women with dramatic illness seemed to me more memorable because women in this age group are usually supporters rather than sufferers, bringing children and elderly relatives to see the doctor but seldom coming for themselves.

In early 1983 in Glasgow, I gave a paper on Down's syndrome at a meeting and, on the same programme, Ken Fegan, a physician in West Kilbride and a former school acquaintance, gave a paper on his research on people in his practice with myalgic encephalomyelitis or chronic fatigue syndrome (Fegan et al., 1983). I can honestly say that this was the first time I had ever heard the term. Later that year I came to New Zealand as the first Professor of General Practice in the country. When I arrived, there was widespread controversy about the Otago outbreak of what was called Tapanui flu, after the town in West Otago where Dr Peter Snow had described many cases (Poore et al., 1984).

Shortly after arriving, I was asked in a press interview whether I thought that Tapanui Flu was a real disease, whatever that means, and I replied that I thought it was. That was when the persons started to come and tell the individual stories of their lives falling apart. From that point on, I became involved in documenting the factual reality of many hundreds of sick people whose lives had fallen apart and whose symptoms corresponded with the criteria of CFS.

Between 1983 and 1992 I was able to document the clinical records of over 400 people who consulted me in my family practice and in whom I made a diagnosis of ME syndrome, later to be called CFS. In these clinical records is recorded the story of their illness, what seemed to be the trigger for it and the length of time spent in getting a diagnosis. A further 100–150 people with fatiguing illnesses also consulted me but I felt unable to make this diagnosis. These other people either had diagnoses which gave a better explanation of their problems or there was no current explanation for their problems. Other studies which have been used are those of the laboratory findings in 200 people (Murdoch, 1987), the symptoms and social problems in 70 people, the psychiatric and personality profiles in 58 people, comparing them with age and sex-matched controls and chronic pain patients (Blakely et al., 1991), a study of cell-mediated immunity in 32 patients and controls (Murdoch, 1988b) and a study of red-cell shape in 69 people (Simpson et al., 1993). Information about the usefulness of professionals and treatments was also collected from a group of 131 people seen between 1984 and 1988 (Murdoch, 1995). The clinical views which I hold are therefore based on observations made during contact with approximately 1000 people, all of whom lived in New Zealand and most of whom lived in the south of New Zealand. There was an overlap of about 200 within this 1000 people, so we are looking at the individual experience of about 800 people.

In the authorship of this book, however, there is also a unique story in that the two authors first met when HDP consulted me regarding her illness and that of her two children that I diagnosed as being CFS. After her recovery from CFS, HDP became a research assistant in the Department of General Practice at the Dunedin School of Medicine of which I was Professor and Chair. She went on to do her own independent research on CFS and other areas and gained her PhD at the University of Otago in 1996. Thus, the most important insights in this book arise directly from the patient–doctor relationship.'

Whatever happened to Wendy Jones?

Wendy's illness probably came on quite suddenly but it would have taken a few days or weeks for her to become a patient or a case. Such issues usually come to the attention of the medical system in a consultation with the person's doctor but the decision to talk about it at all will depend on many factors. On the patient's side there is usually a decision to be made on what is 'normal' with respect to symptoms such as tiredness and people will say, 'I really feel tired', or 'I should not be this tired'. We suspect that leading with the symptom of tiredness is probably because it is such a familiar symptom. It is difficult in most cultures to admit that life is falling apart, which would be nearer the truth. Often, other family members will have been consulted and their reaction might depend on their experience of the person complaining or of the family's track record in tiredness. 'Oh you're always tired', or 'That's interesting; Uncle Fred was this tired last year before he was diagnosed with cancer', might be the content of these family consultations.

The appointment is then made with the doctor so that the symptoms can be further evaluated. It is often assumed that physicians use a standard approach to the patients who consult them. However, the research which has been done, mainly by doctors themselves, shows that there can be a vast difference in the ways in which such complex symptoms are assessed. The two main approaches are to quickly screen the problems presented by the patient using either a doctor-centered or a patient-centered approach. It is important to understand that in most places the emphasis in primary care is on a brief evaluation. In the UK, where access to the doctor is 'free of charge', the average time for each consultation is six minutes, whereas in other countries where payment has to be made for access, the patient may have a longer consultation. However, even there the trend seems to be that general practitioners prefer shorter consultations and the average time is not much longer, probably 10 minutes.

The doctor-centered approach

Going to a doctor who uses the doctor-centered approach is a bit like going to a government office to fill in a form for a benefit or a service. The doctor asks all the questions and the answers which the patient gives are usually of the yes/no variety. One of the problems in this evaluation is that, in the case of complicated 'falling apart' episodes such as Wendy's, it is difficult in the short time available to get through all the symptoms. In addition, the numerous symptoms are entirely subjective, and they sound a bit silly as they are coming out. Because she knows that the doctor is looking for certain diagnoses she may be tempted to answer these selectively and she will probably not emphasize anything which might lead him to conclude that she has a nervous or emotional problem. However, most doctors will proceed to ask systematically about other symptoms, other diseases already experienced and relevant family history. The liturgy of this was taught to all doctors at medical school and it is fairly standard. There are some external tests to differentiate between mild and severe tiredness but most doctors prefer to talk with the patient and make up their minds as to whether the complaint should be taken seriously according to these standard questions. Many patients with CFS find that the doctor shows signs of not taking things seriously in the first interview. From doctor to doctor there seems to be little standardization of the meaning of such reported symptoms and the patient's word and the doctor's previous experience seem to be the only arbiters. One of the really valuable aspects of continuity of care is that, over time, the same doctor can evaluate such subjective symptoms with the same patient, but, as we can see with Dr Rose, a previously unblemished record does not seem to compensate for a poor present performance.

If the doctor feels it is warranted, the patient will then be asked to lie down and the doctor will carry out a physical examination based on the symptoms complained of. During this examination the only clue that something is abnormal is when the doctor takes a long time about a particular aspect of the examination. He/she will then suggest that the person has a few investigations, which again depend on the associated symptoms. In a case like Wendy's, there is usually no immediate feedback and when she gets back home and Willie asks her 'Well, what did the doctor say/think?', she will reply that he asked a few questions, gave her a full examination and sent off some blood for some tests. He also asked her to come back a week later to discuss the results.

In the doctor-centered consultation this follow-up visit is the key to whether you have won or lost the battle for the doctor's attention. Usually the tiredness is only taken seriously if the search for a cause reveals some underlying problem which the doctor recognizes as important. For example, if Dr Rose had taken a blood test that revealed that Wendy was suffering from acute leukemia, she would immediately have been taken seriously. He would have referred her to a consultant hematologist or oncologist and by now would be undergoing treatment. Although her husband and parents would be extremely worried about her, they would also be extremely sympathetic and there would be a definite plan or treatment and support available to the family. If she had died, Dr Rose would be heartily thanked for his care and attention.

She did not die but the relationship between her and Dr Rose is moribund for reasons much simpler than the complexity of her illness. The first is the failure of communication. Her first consultation with him was six months ago when her unasked question was 'What is going on? Why am I so tired?', and he still has not answered her. He could have told her that he did not know, which would have been the accurate and compassionate answer, but he has said nothing. According to the doctor and diagnosis-centered philosophy he does not have to answer unless he has something to say. No news is not good news, it is no news.

The second problem is that Dr Rose is a good doctor only when his patients have something wrong with them that he can diagnose and treat. His care and attention come with conditions that Wendy cannot fulfill. Unless she has an abnormal blood test or X-ray she cannot be accepted as a person who can be helped. This conditional approach betrays some very old-fashioned, but dearly held beliefs in the medical community and the community at large concerning who is eligible for the attention of the health system and its social supports. Patients and doctors still assume that illness must have a specific cause or alternatively be a readily recognizable disease and that, if no cause is found, then the person cannot really be ill. Where the doctor-centered approach assumes that a cause can be found for every common symptom, it has been proved wrong. Research in primary care (McWhinney, 1984) has shown that this assumption is false about two-thirds of the time on average, even where the complaint is more specific, like chest pain, abdominal pain or headache. Thus, people like Wendy whose physical examination and blood tests are within the normal range are assumed to be physically well, with disastrous effects on their suffering. This situation is not improving because as orthodox medical care becomes more expensive these very criteria are now used to decide which illnesses are treated through government or insurer and which are not. It is our impression that many people now seek care through alternative medicine because they do not have the diseases that qualify them to attend medical doctors.

All this is bad enough but there is worse to come. In the old days people could attend doctors and be given a placebo, or a hug, or both. Although doctors concentrated on looking for a *hall of fame* diagnosis, there was so much uncertainty because of the lack of diagnostic tests, such as ultrasound and CAT scans, that they had to be prepared to find a place for uncertainty. There was also a paternalistic sense of ownership of patients that meant that people received some sort of management irrespective of the symptoms. Now doctors like Dr Rose have become obsessed with being clinically and politically correct (medically speaking) and the result is that they believe that people like Wendy are pretending to be ill or to have some delusion that they are ill. There are even forms that she can fill in which will demonstrate all this. Every time she meets the doctor the message is reinforced and a wall is erected between her and her doctor. It seems that the only door through this wall is diagnosis and the list of accepted diagnoses is firmly in the hands of the doctor. At the heart of the problem is a philosophical and an attitudinal aspect to the doctor–patient interaction. Both doctor and patient would prefer to find a cause for the problem and are both still embarrassed, hurt or ashamed when no such outcome is forthcoming.

8 Chronic fatigue syndrome: a patient-centered approach

In the simplest of consultations there is great relief on both sides when a cause is found.

Patient: I have a sore throat.
Doctor: The throat is very inflamed with flecks of yellow pus.
Patient: What is wrong with me?
Doctor: You have tonsillitis and here are some antibiotics. You will be better in a few days.

Such a scenario makes life very simple for both patient and doctor but in the 20 to 40 consultations which a doctor has every day, only about three are in that category.

The doctor- or diagnosis-centered approach has some very significant weaknesses in the management of illness generally and these are not confined to people like Wendy whose illnesses are vague and unrecognized. The same inflexibility of approach has led to a change of philosophy in other more specific areas such as the immediate care of acutely injured people, palliative care of the dying, care of the elderly and the intellectually handicapped. In the case of care of the acutely injured this doctor- and diagnosis-centered approach was costing lives.

The approach to the injured patient, as being taught in medical schools, was the same as that for a patient with a previously undiagnosed medical condition, i.e. an extensive history including past medical history, a physical examination starting at the top of the head and progressing down the body, and finally the development of a differential diagnosis and a list of adjuncts to confirm the diagnosis. Although this approach was quite adequate for a patient with diabetes mellitus or even many acute surgical illnesses, it did not satisfy the needs of the patient suffering life-threatening injury. (American College of Surgeons, 1997)

The story behind the development of what is now called Advanced Trauma Life Support (ATLS) was the realization that doctors wasted so much time on the pursuit of accurate diagnosis in such situations, that the patients died as they puzzled. The solution was to retrain them in what is known as immediate care.

In the philosophy of ATLS (1997) there are three important underlying concepts. These are:

1 Treat the greatest threat to life first
2 Don't let the lack of a definitive diagnosis impede the application of an indicated treatment
3 A detailed history is not necessary to begin the evaluation.

Simple and easily remembered principles were introduced, such as:

1. Airway with cervical spine protection
2. Breathing
3. Circulation-control external bleeding
4. Disability or neurological status
5. Exposure (undress) and Environment (temperature control).

Such has been the influence of the immediate care movement to the management of the acutely injured patient that any doctor who did not now follow these principles would be regarded as dangerous and the ambulance services and police would ask for a replacement doctor and report him or her to the disciplinary body for doctors.

> So here is the question to assess how Dr Rose is doing in appropriate immediate care.
> As the doctor on duty, you are called out to an emergency on the local highway. There has been a head-on collision by a motorist into the concrete pillar of a bridge. When you arrive the fire and ambulance personnel have located the badly injured driver hanging upside down in the cab with her legs trapped by the steering wheel. There is a hysterical passenger in the front seat and a baby and a little boy luckily well strapped in the back seat. Do you:
>
> - take a full history and physical from the driver, arrange a few blood tests and ask her to see you next week?
> - insist that before the driver is removed from the car, a full investigation of the cause of the accident should be completed?
> - ask the driver and the passenger to complete a General Health Questionnaire and label them as psychiatric cases?
> - suggest that the accident might never have happened if the couple had organized their life better?

You may think that these questions are all ridiculous, but Dr Alan Rose's approach to Wendy's problem is not all that different. She has crashed her life and in doing so has done great damage to the health and welfare of herself, her husband and her children. The doctor who has been called to the scene is just as dangerous and ineffective as the untrained bumbler at the scene of the accident. In her case, his demanding a cause is just as dangerous because the longer he keeps telling her that there is nothing wrong, the more her life and the lives of those she loves and cares for fall apart. What is required is the equivalent of immediate care for this person whose life has fallen apart and the principles are very similar.

1 What is the greatest threat here?
2 Don't let the lack of a definitive diagnosis impede the application of an indicated treatment.
3 A detailed history is not necessary to begin the evaluation.

The person-centered approach

This provides a better way to focus immediate care for these severely traumatized people. This method affirms that Wendy is the central character in the drama, the only person who can tell us which symptoms are present, who can comment on their quality and their effect on her everyday function. According to this model (Levenstein *et al.*,1986; Stewart *et al.*, 1995), each new episode of illness has never happened quite this way before and the doctor who disbelieves or distrusts the patient misses a golden opportunity to measure the extent and the quality of the symptoms.

When a person like Wendy pops up the doctor is really struggling to understand just what has happened precisely because her experience is unique. The answer, therefore, is not to try to match the symptoms and signs to something in a textbook, but to remain open to the narrative produced by Wendy and to try to find parallels within the catalogues of professional and personal experience that can be helpful in making her experience a little more bearable. Even when this is not possible, the doctor can use his or her past experience of that person to help with the struggle.

There should be three clear phases to this sort of consultation and attention to these helps to extend the possibilities in diagnosis.

1 **Recognition of the suffering.** This is the immediate care that is needed by people like Wendy. It is the ABC. It is as if we go to the crashed wreck of a life and say 'Hello in there, are you okay?' The words can never be learned off pat but all that was required to be said by Dr Rose here was 'Wendy, this is not like you. I can see that your life has fallen apart'. He was the doctor who had been seeing her and her family for some years. He had shared her ante-natal care, delivered the baby and knew her medical history. Yet he omitted to acknowledge the extent of her current suffering and without that witness he seemed cold and aloof. The first mark of a true healer is the perception of the state which needs to be healed and the expression of concern which is unconditional.
2 **Diagnostic search for a cause.** There are many possible reasons for tiredness especially in a lactating mother. Few of these are diagnosed by blood tests. She may be anemic, she may be depressed, she may simply be exhausted by the amount she has to do. Being patient-centered involves just as much

diagnostic acumen on the part of the doctor as being doctor-centered. However, the agenda is shared and at each point the doctor discusses with the patient her or his view on the possibilities of diagnosis. This means that the healing can start before embarking on the search for a cause, and means that the time spent in searching is not wasted.

3 **Naming and explanation**. This is the springboard for healing and most people are happier with a name for their problem. Along with the name come a set of criteria which all such cases have in common and with them comes an opportunity to make generalizations about how the illness behaves, how long it lasts and how the person can be healed.

Evolution of the criteria for chronic fatigue syndrome

Our present criteria for CFS have arisen directly from the information collected during person-centered consultations. After many years of discussion a consensus has emerged from various parts of the world on exactly which symptoms should be included in the syndrome, and this has come about as people have told doctors about their illnesses. This has resulted in the consensus of an internationally recognized definition and the result is that recognition can be easier for the next person who comes along. Wendy can be categorized as a case rather than a mystery. The agreement on who is a case has been surprisingly easy, much easier than gaining agreement on how she should be treated. As a result of this process we now know that the illness from which she suffers is CFS.

In 1988 the Center for Communicable Disease (Holmes *et al.*, 1988) produced a working case definition of CFS which was modified in 1994 in the light of further discussion (Fukuda *et al.*, 1994). This definition became accepted as the international definition although it was mainly used in the US. There were two main criteria:

- Clinically evaluated, unexplained, persistent or relapsing chronic fatigue that is of new or definite onset (i.e. is not lifelong), is not the result of on-going exertion, is not substantially alleviated by rest and results in substantial reduction in previous levels of occupational, educational, social or personal activities
- The concurrent occurrence of four or more of the following symptoms:
  - substantial impairment of short-term memory or concentration
  - sore throat
  - tender lymph nodes

- muscle pain
- multi-joint pain without swelling or redness
- headaches of a new type, pattern or severity
- unrefreshing sleep
- post-exertional malaise lasting more than 24 hours.

In addition, the case definition asks the doctor to identify conditions which make this diagnosis impossible (because they have a diagnosis which would also explain the symptoms).

- Any active medical condition that may explain chronic fatigue such as an underactive thyroid, sleep apnea and narcolepsy and side effects of medication.
- If the patient has had a diagnosis before, such as cancer or a chronic infection like hepatitis B or C, because the present illness might be a relapse of the original one.
- Any past or present diagnosis of major psychiatric illness such as bipolar affective disorder (manic-depressive psychosis), schizophrenia, dementia, anorexia or bulimia.
- Alcohol or substance abuse occurring within two years of the onset of chronic fatigue.
- Severe obesity with a body mass index of 45 or greater, i.e. a woman of 170 cm who weighs 130 kg or a man of 180 cm who weighs 145 kg.

There are some minor concerns about this definition, mainly that it still retains a link to glandular fever or Epstein–Barr virus infection, and sore throat and tender lymph nodes are not necessarily common in CFS. However, the criteria are similar to those that have been suggested by groups in other countries.

In New Zealand in 1986, the Mackenzie Foundation (Murdoch, 1988a) funded a series of meetings in which representatives of consumers, health professionals and medical researchers came together to discuss the criteria for diagnosis for what they agreed to call ME syndrome. These Mackenzie criteria were:

- an illness duration of greater than six months
- symptoms that should include chronic fatigue, muscle pain and early muscle weakness after exercise
- a relapsing course
- age inclusion of 16 to 60 years.

In Australia (Lloyd *et al.*, 1988) the definition used was developed by the team of researchers working in the University of New South Wales and has the following criteria:

- Chronic persisting or relapsing fatigue of a generalized nature, exacerbated by minor exercise, causing significant disruption of usual daily activities and present for greater than six months
- Neuropsychiatric dysfunction, including impairment of concentration evidenced by difficulty in completing mental tasks which were easily accomplished before the onset of the syndrome and new onset of short-term memory impairment
- No alternative diagnosis reached by history, physical examination or investigation over a six month period.

In the UK in 1990, a group of experts devised the Oxford Criteria (Sharpe et al., 1991) which defined CFS as a syndrome characterized by:

- a definite onset that is not lifelong
- fatigue as the principal symptom
- fatigue which is severe, disabling and affects both physical and mental functioning
- fatigue which has been present for a minimum of six months during which it was present more than 50% of the time
- other symptoms that may be present, particularly myalgia, mood and sleep disturbances.

Specific exclusion criteria included:

- an established medical condition known to produce severe fatigue
- a current diagnosis of schizophrenia, manic depression, substance abuse, eating disorder or proven organic brain disease.

These sets of criteria are all very similar to each other and provide an important basis for allowing people to be seen in a classification which allows them to have a named illness and for us to be able to agree on the prevalence of the illness in various populations. Apart from the New Zealand criteria, they have largely been the result of discussions between doctors and patients and it is important that they be regarded as statements of the common-reported experience of persons affected, rather than another form which patients have to complete to qualify for the illness.

Evaluating Wendy: keep it simple, Dr Rose

These then are the criteria and an evaluation can be done by consulting a properly trained family physician, general practitioner or general internist. It is very important that this should be done in consultation with a primary care physician as there are so many different conditions that can cause fatigue. After a careful history and physical examination to exclude the common exclusions given above, the patient should have a screen of basic laboratory investigations (Komaroff and Buchwald, 1998), such as:

- examination of the urine
- full blood count
- erythrocyte sedimentation rate
- anti-nuclear antigen
- fasting morning cortisol
- serum immunoglobulins
- tuberculosis testing
- lyme serology
- HIV testing.

Some of these tests will only be justified where the patients' circumstances indicate it, but it is emphasized that this should be the maximum testing done in primary care. If no other positive diagnosis has been made within the six month timeframe, and the symptoms specified in the CDC definition are there, then the illness should be labelled as CFS.

However, within a month of her developing these symptoms, and depending on the result of the evaluation, it could have been established that Wendy was suffering from presumed CFS and there is great value in doing this. After six months she should be told that she is suffering from definite CFS if she has symptoms of headache, pains in her muscles, sleep disturbance and memory loss. If she has not had that typical pattern of symptoms and there is no other definitive diagnosis, she could have been told that she had idiopathic chronic fatigue (ICF).

So what was the problem with Dr Rose doing this? The real problem was that Dr Rose was well behind the times and had not kept up with the international literature on the subject.

The importance of naming the illness

It is impossible to overemphasize the sense of relief that results when a person is given a name for their illness (Wood, 1991). CFS has been called the 'disease of a thousand names' and, indeed, it has been called many things in different parts of the world. Many, particularly patients, believe 'chronic fatigue syndrome' is an inadequate term because, as we have already said, it fails to describe adequately the range of the characteristic symptoms and the severity of fatigue.

For that reason, in New Zealand we preferred the term 'ME syndrome'. However, most medical authorities seem to prefer the term 'chronic fatigue syndrome' because it is descriptive and free from unproven claims with respect to causation. The name myalgic encephalomyelitis (ME) suggests that there is inflammation in the brain and spinal cord, which is not present, and that of chronic fatigue and immunodeficiency syndrome (CFIDS) suggests that all have immunodeficiency, which is also incorrect.

The important thing is that we now have a name and that name, whatever it is, breaks the isolation of illness and its use indicates that doctors recognize the illness and its common criteria. The naming also makes the problem much easier to handle. In his classic book about a country doctor in England, John Berger (1967) wrote:

> Patients are inordinately relieved when doctors give their complaint a name. The name may mean very little to them; they may understand nothing of what it signifies; but because it has a name, it has an independent existence from them. They can now struggle or complain against it. To have a complaint recognized, that is to say defined, limited and depersonalized, is to be made stronger.

Berger was writing in the 1960s when few doctors were prepared to give their patients the name of CFS for their illness. Indeed, the breakthrough in the 1980s has been that patients have decided to name their own illness, although, admittedly with the help of a few doctors who were prepared to make a study of the illness. The same relief comes when they are given the name either through taking it themselves or through joining a support group. In the case of CFS this has produced a problem because some patients diagnose themselves before consulting doctors, and it may be difficult to persuade them that it is some other problem such as undiagnosed cancer or multiple sclerosis or depression which is the cause of their fatiguing illness. However, the dangers of this inappropriate naming are far less than the isolation experienced by Wendy and the subsequent blaming of her which has led to considerable family difficulty.

However, it is also important that the name has clinical meaning. There is a distinct difference between the terms CFS, prolonged fatigue and ICF, and it is important that everyone dealing with people whose lives have been affected by unusual tiredness are aware of just how valuable it is to use the precise name. To tell someone nothing or to say ' I don't know what it is, but you've got it' is not helpful. It is particularly important that general practitioners and other doctors working in primary care should be up to date with these different manifestations of fatigue. Most people with this problem will present in primary care and the evidence seems to suggest that those in whom the criteria for CFS are not present are usually told that they suffer from nothing rather than a diagnosis such as prolonged fatigue or ICF.

Estimating the prevalence of chronic fatigue syndrome

The great advantage of having internationally agreed criteria for fatigue, chronic fatigue and CFS is that we can compare the number of people who are thus affected in various parts of the world. It must be remembered that the definition of CFS is an agreed description of the key symptoms and that there is still no agreement on what causes the person to have these symptoms. There is also no final agreement on whether there is necessarily a relationship between CFS and prolonged or chronic fatigue. The adoption of the criteria for CFS has allowed us to emphasize the important differences between CFS and fatigue: simple, prolonged or chronic.

Fatigue is a very common symptom in the community and in attenders in primary care. The prevalence of fatigue has been reported as 32% of consecutive consulting patients in the US (Bates et al., 1993) and in up to 45% of females in both community and primary care studies (Lewis and Wessely, 1992). In an Australian study in primary care, 25% of 1593 patients had fatigue of at least two weeks duration and, of these, two-thirds were also classified as cases of psychological disorder using the General Health Questionnaire (Hickie et al., 1996). Those who had fatigue were more likely to be female, of lower socioeconomic status and had less years of formal education. In a larger UK study, a postal questionnaire to 15 283 men and women aged 18–45 revealed that 38% suffered from substantial fatigue as revealed through a validated fatigue scale (Pawlikowska et al., 1994). Again there was a higher prevalence in women and an association with psychological distress. Using the same translated instrument, the prevalence of substantial fatigue in a population of attenders at a physician's clinic in the United Arab Emirates (UAE) was 64.8% compared with 10% in Western studies, with 70.4% of patients having fatigue (McIlvenny, 1998). The duration of their fatigue varied from one day to 45 years with a mean duration of three years. In only 3% of these consultations was fatigue noted by the doctor. The most recent community-based study has shown that 7.7% of a large community sample suffered from prolonged fatigue (Jason et al., 1999).

Chronic fatigue differs only from fatigue or prolonged fatigue in lasting longer and is, not surprisingly, less common. In the British study quoted above (Pawlikowska et al., 1994) the prevalence of chronic fatigue was 18.3%. In a study of 2376 subjects, aged 18–45 years (Wessely et al. 1997), the point prevalence of chronic fatigue was 11.3%, falling to 4.1% if co-morbid psychological disorders were excluded. Rates did not vary by social class. After adjustment for psychological disorder, being female was only modestly associated with chronic fatigue. Functional impairment was profound and was associated with psychological disorder. In the UAE study the figure was 44.8%. Another study in the

US (Buchwald *et al.*, 1995) observed that the prevalence of chronic fatigue was 19.2% in a random sample of members of a health maintenance organization. In this study two-thirds of the 590 people with chronic fatigue had some physical or psychiatric illness as a reason for their chronic fatigue. They found no sex or minority group difference in those with chronic fatigue. A community-based study in Chicago (Jason *et al.*, 1999) found a prevalence of 4.2% for chronic fatigue.

Because of the lack of agreement over criteria, the prevalence of CFS has always been difficult to estimate. The illness which has these agreed criteria has been occurring in outbreaks for the past 60 years and individual reports have been very similar to those given by Wendy (*see* Chapter 3). It is difficult to categorize these retrospectively but it would seem that the prevalence in the population was quite high, e.g. in the outbreak reported by Fegan *et al.* (1983) in the West of Scotland, the prevalence was 488 per 100 000, and in another (Keighley and Bell, 1983) was 680 per 100 000. The first attempt at estimating the prevalence in New Zealand was in West Otago (Poore *et al.*, 1984). Retrospectively the CDC criteria have been applied to 23 of the 28 cases described and 10 were confirmed as CFS, a prevalence of 200 per 100 000 (Levine *et al.*, 1997). Another attempt at prevalence based on the Mackenzie criteria and on individuals seen in Dunedin was 127 per 100 000 (Murdoch, 1987). A survey of a geographically stratified sample of 149 of the 2000 family physicians in New Zealand in 1984 found that they could recall 172 people with ME-like symptoms lasting two months or more. This approximated to a prevalence of 72 per 100 000 (Royal New Zealand College of General Practitioners, 1985).

These attempts at estimating the prevalence of CFS were the result of dramatic symptoms occurring in patients and being noted by their doctors. As the event producing the observation was not standardized by an agreed definition, many of these studies have been dismissed as exaggeration. However, this may well be a more reliable way of estimating the prevalence of CFS than was first realized. A further study of 98 Otago general practitioners (Denz-Penhey and Murdoch, 1993) showed a minimum prevalence rate of 167 per 100 000. Another study in Scotland (Ho-Yen and Macnamara, 1991) had a much higher prevalence of 1300 per 100 000. If the West Otago re-categorization (Levine *et al.*, 1997) is a guide, it would appear that around 50% could have been wrongly classified as CFS. However, Jason's community study in Chicago described overleaf revealed that only 50% of people sought medical help for CFS and so any over inclusion could well be compensated for by under-reporting.

Most countries have experienced an intense political furore surrounding the recognition of CFS, with patients wishing to receive support and doctors resisting the diagnosis. Early attempts to counter the fear that communities were facing a public health hazard resulted in the estimation of some extremely low prevalence rates precisely because they depended on doctors being willing to recognize CFS. There are clear indications that there is great variation in such recognition. In the 1984 New Zealand family physician survey, 56% accepted ME as a diagnostic entity while 71% of Scottish family physicians accepted the diagnosis of CFS in 1993 (Ho-Yen and Macnamara, 1991). A survey of Otago general practitioners in 1993 (Denz-Penhey and Murdoch, 1993) showed that 93% accepted CFS as a diagnosis. Whether this change was brought about by the change of name or the introduction of criteria is unclear. Also, clusters of patients could afford to travel to consult 'experts' and this tended to overestimate the prevalence by multiple counting of the same cases. This early clustering around interested doctors which occurred in most countries also produced confounding opinions about CFS, such as that it was more common in 'yuppies' and that professional health workers were being selectively affected, but more formal studies have failed to confirm these early opinions (Wessely *et al.*, 1997).

In the US, the Centers for Disease Control set up a surveillance study in response to political pressure from CFS support groups. In this study patients were enrolled by physicians in four US cities and this produced what is now regarded as the very low figure of 2.7 per 100 000 (Gunn *et al.*, 1993). A population-based study in Australia using notification from local general practitioners estimated the prevalence to be 37.1 per 100 000 (Lloyd *et al.*, 1990). In the UK where general practitioners care for defined populations the estimates of prevalence have been much higher. Wessely and his colleagues (1997) found a prevalence of 800 to 1800 per 100 000 in a population of 2376 seen in general practices and another study (Lawrie *et al.*, 1997) in a single practice estimated a prevalence of 600 per 100 000. A further study in the Pacific North-west of the US estimated the prevalence to range between 17–267 cases per 100 000 (Buchwald *et al.*, 1995).

The marked variation in the prevalence of CFS in these studies could be understood as being a treatment bias, i.e. they were done by physicians with the power to attract patients through their specializing in the subject and who use the CFS criteria to qualify people for the diagnosis. However, as has already been seen in the case of Wendy, any doctor has the power to make a person a case or to refuse such a diagnosis. In addition, there may be many people in the community who have the symptoms of CFS but who have not consulted physicians. This possibility was answered by a comprehensive community-based study in Chicago (Jason *et al.*, 1999) which suggested that some of the previous estimates of prevalence had been conservative. In this study of 28 673 individuals, the overall prevalence was 420 per 100 000. However, while confirming a greater prevalence in females (522 vs 291) the study also showed that the highest prevalence was in Latino groups at 726, with African Americans at 337 and Whites at 318. The most commonly affected age group was 40–49 with a prevalence of 805 per 100 000. Skilled workers were the most commonly affected occupational group (701), with unskilled workers at 486 and professionals at 325. This refutes earlier claims that the most commonly affected group were young, upwardly mobile professionals. The study confirmed a high association with psychiatric disorder and when CFS cases were compared to controls they were more likely to be unemployed, in part-time work and on disability incomes.

These most recent studies tell us that, while CFS is fortunately much less common than chronic fatigue and prolonged fatigue, it is certainly a diagnosis which has to be remembered as a possibility in primary care. In fact, the authors of the Chicago study make the point that it is a very common women's health problem, being well ahead of HIV infection (12/100 000), multiple sclerosis (70), breast cancer (26), lung cancer (33), and is only outstripped by diabetes (900), hypertension (3000) heart disease (3400) and arthritis (3800). It is certainly much more common than a spontaneous pneumothorax, subarachnoid hemorrhage or nephrotic syndrome. Any doctor who missed any of these diagnoses would be subject to scrutiny as to competence to practice. However, it is the all too common complaint of CFS sufferers that, like Wendy, they are left ignorant of the possibility that they have CFS. The fact that Jason's study revealed a prevalence 100 times greater than that of the CDC study seems to suggest that some doctors are still blind to the possibility of this diagnosis.

One explanation for this underestimate is that it became forgotten that one of the problems in estimating prevalence is that this will vary not only with the definition but also with the ability of those who are counting to recognize the symptoms and place them in the context of a separate disorder. The various definitions arose as the response of those who needed to give a specific diagnosis to the people with the symptoms who presented to them. There were other doctors who believed that existing diagnoses, such as fibromyalgia syndrome, mitral valve prolapse, depression or somatoform disorder were appropriate and labelled their patients accordingly. However, the vast majority of doctors, and therefore patients, will be like Dr Rose and Wendy and will be pronounced as having no diagnosis. Such epidemiological dyslexia has bedevilled attempts to find the true prevalence of CFS.

The discipline of accurately describing chronic fatigue syndrome

The great advantage of having agreed international criteria for CFS is that these allow us to map and study a disorder which is distinct from fatigue and chronic fatigue but whose etiology is as yet unknown. There is little compelling evidence that CFS is necessarily related to prolonged or chronic fatigue, as any actual observer of the person at the beginning of this illness would know. The difference is more than the semantic necessity to wait six months before being allowed to call the illness CFS. The argument proposed by those who link the disorders implies that, if Wendy developed the illness on 1st October, it would be 'fatigue' until the 1st of November, 'chronic fatigue' until the 1st of April when, on an appropriate date, it would become CFS. However, to qualify as a case of CFS, Wendy has to have the criteria of CFS from day one.

If she had been tired with her worry about the kids and the stresses of Willie's new business, she would have had fatigue. This is a universal phenomenon but for most of us the important issue is that within a few hours we feel better again. If she had felt tired for a week or more, she may have begun to try and rationalize it and might have set in train her own solutions, such as having an early night or laying off the food or alcohol. If that hadn't worked, she would have asked around and eventually she might have ended up consulting her doctor. The assumption we might gain from the literature is that CFS is chronic fatigue, only worse, but Wendy's experience is that this problem was bad from the beginning. Her life fell apart and she developed the specific symptoms contained in the criteria.

The largely self-appointed group of experts whose names appear on these agreements are always, however, in danger of breaking ranks and using these agreements to argue theories of causation. A good example of this is the increasing tendency to return to the explanation (McEvedy and Beard, 1970) of CFS as a 'functional somatic syndrome' (Wessely et al., 1999). This theory of causation is greatly aided by discussing CFS in the context of fatigue and chronic fatigue, even neurasthenia. (Hickie et al., 1997). However, the purpose of the criteria is to describe the entity of CFS and not to argue for a particular causation. The concept of functional or psychosomatic disorders is a defendable one, as we shall see in Chapter 3. However, the problem with this concept is that it appears to deny that any cause will ever be found. This is because the term 'functional' means *having no discernable organic cause* and the term 'psychosomatic' means *caused or aggravated by mental conflict or stress*. The tendency to regard CFS as a subset of chronic fatigue, which in turn is a subset of fatigue, while attractive intellectually, by placing CFS in a certain context is no more logical than that of regarding multiple sclerosis or rheumatoid arthritis, both of which have fatigue as a predominant symptom, as subsets of fatigue. These disputes about causation seem to arise from the failure to recognize that all significant illnesses are multilevel disorders involving bodily functioning, emotions and social relationships (Epstein et al., 1999).

However, many papers discuss both conditions together, giving the impression that CFS somehow springs from CF (Bombardier and Buchwald, 1995; Hartz et al., 1999) or that a study on fatigued patients provides information on CFS even when less than 2% of those with fatigue attribute it to CFS (Pawlikowska et al., 1994). However, in our experience, CFS is a qualitatively different issue which involves a *crash* – a dramatic appearance of the inability to maintain even 50% of normal activities through:

Clinically evaluated, unexplained, persistent or relapsing chronic fatigue that is of new or definite onset (i.e. is not lifelong), is not the result of on-going exertion, is not substantially alleviated by rest, and results in substantial reduction in previous levels of occupational, educational, social or personal activities

with the addition of four or more of the symptoms mentioned above (Fukuda et al., 1994).

The spirit of this operational definition is its use in people like Wendy during the first six months of the illness in order to reduce the level of physical, psychological and social disability that is produced. We find it difficult to understand how this kind of definition can be applied to large populations of people who have not been observed developing the illness in the timeframe of six months. Jason et al. made this criticism of the studies which found a high 'paper' prevalence of CFS in the UK (Lawrie et al., 1997; Wessely et al., 1997), but it must be remembered that the Chicago study is based on the findings in 166 out of 408 people who were found to have CFS-like findings. Of this physician-screened sample 89 (54%) had medical or psychiatric reasons for their illness, 45 (27%) had none of the criteria of CFS and 32 (19%) had CFS. Thus, it is likely that the British studies quoted above may have overestimated the prevalence of CFS by as much as a factor of 5, bringing the prevalence back somewhere between 100–500 per 100 000. Thus, the prevalence rates quoted above drawing on the memory of family physicians and the dramas of their patients may not have been as wide off the mark as first thought.

A final point is that these are measures of prevalence and not incidence. To return to our immediate care parallel, there is a difference between a car crash with the victims still inside and a wrecked car safe in a layby and waiting to be towed to a service station. The personal stories of people with CFS as related to their own doctors will be the only means of calculating a true incidence for the condition. Perhaps the accuracy of the prevalence figures reached by the personal witness of family doctors will encourage us to use a more patient-centered approach to our research.

The natural history of defined chronic fatigue syndrome

Another great advantage of having an agreed operational definition for CFS is that studies can be done which tell us what the course of the illness is likely to be. When a person consults a physician the most important question after 'What is wrong with me?' is ' How long is it going to last?'

One of the problems in providing such information is that the answer to this question seems to vary according to the group studied in the first place. Much of the information collected about groups of people with CFS comes from the collaboration of patient-support groups with medical *centers of excellence* usually based in tertiary hospitals. This inevitably produces a bias towards severity because it is a simple fact that those who are severely ill and do not recover will be more noticed than those who are ill and then recover.

Until more light is shed on the possible causes of CFS, it will be impossible to give a clear answer to this question. Most follow-up studies done from CFS clinics give a pessimistic view. A Dutch study (Vercoulen et al., 1996) reported that only 3% of 246 people had recovered after 18 months, 17% had improved and 20% were worse. An Australian study (Wilson et al., 1994) reported that 6% of 103 people had recovered but that 57% had improved. A follow up to a British study (Bonner et al., 1994) showed that 16 of 29 (55%) people diagnosed as having CFS and given treatment had improved four years later. A review of the literature (Joyce et al., 1997) of the studies on outcome published to that point showed that the outlook in adults with CFS was poor, with less than 10% returning to what they were like before the illness and the remainder being significantly impaired. The factors which associated with poor prognosis were older age, more chronic illness, having a co-morbid psychiatric disorder and holding a belief that the illness is due to physical causes. In children the prognosis was much better, with 54%–94% recovered over the period of follow-up.

However, there are indications that where the problem is studied in primary care, the outcome seems more optimistic. A follow-up of the patients affected in the West Otago study (Levine et al., 1997) showed that a high proportion (75%) had returned to the level of health that they had before the illness. In an unpublished questionnaire study (Murdoch, 1995) 131 individuals in whom JCM had made a diagnosis of MES were followed up a minimum of a year later and asked about their current state of health. Fifteen (12%) of the respondents were totally cured and 87 (66%) much better when compared with what they felt at the start of the illness. Only four (3%) felt worse and three (2%) much worse.

Conclusion

The world is full of people like Wendy Jones and it seems that the most appropriate way for their healthcare needs to be met is to consult with general practitioners or family physicians like Dr Alan Rose. Such doctors look after a population of around 1500 people, of whom 900 will be in the 18–65 age group. This is about one-twentieth of the Chicago sample and, if screened, would reveal only two people with CFS-like symptoms and only one of them would have CFS according to the criteria set out in this chapter. Wendy was only one person but she was ignored by Dr Rose and several people's lives were put at risk by his failure to appreciate what was going on.

CFS is a specific diagnosis that is as different from CF as it is from rheumatoid arthritis or multiple sclerosis. It now has an internationally accepted definition and all that requires to be done is to match the symptoms of the person presenting to the criteria and to label the person appropriately. If this had been done for Wendy she would have had a more appropriate outcome.

Patient-centered care requires immediate care, and the greatest threat to Wendy at this point is her doctor's failure to remember the principles of immediate care.

1 Treat the greatest threat to life first, which is her isolation – the feeling that she is the only one who has ever suffered from this problem. We need to make it clear that we recognize her problem and take it seriously.
2 Don't let the lack of a definitive diagnosis impede the application of an indicated treatment. Even if you cannot bring yourself to call her problem CFS, you could at least call it *CFS-like* or *IFS*.
3 A detailed history is not necessary to begin the evaluation. What is required is the recognition that six months of uncertainty may cause more damage than the risk you may be wrong.

References

American College of Surgeons (1997) *Advanced Trauma Life Support Program for Doctors.* American College of Surgeons, Chicago, IL.

Bates DW, Schmitt W, Buchwald D et al. (1993) Prevalence of fatigue and chronic fatigue syndrome in a primary care practice. *Arch Intern Med.* **153**: 2759–65.

Berger J (1967) *A Fortunate Man: the story of a country doctor.* The Penguin Press, London, UK.

Blakely AA, Howard R, Sosich R et al. (1991) Psychiatric symptoms, personality and ways of coping in chronic fatigue syndrome. *Psychol Med.* **21**: 347–62.

Bombardier CH and Buchwald D (1995) Outcome and prognosis of patients with chronic fatigue vs chronic fatigue syndrome. *Arch Intern Med.* **155**: 2105–10.

Bonner D, Ron M, Chalder T, Butler S and Wessely S (1994) Chronic fatigue syndrome: a follow-up study. *J Neurol Neurosurg Psychiatry.* **57**: 617–21.

Buchwald D, Umali P, Umali J et al. (1995) Chronic fatigue and the chronic fatigue syndrome: prevalence in a Pacific North-west healthcare system. *Arch Intern Med.* **123**: 81–8.

Cox H (1973) *Seduction of the Spirit: the use and misuse of people's religion.* Simon & Schuster, New York.

Denz-Penhey H and Murdoch JC (1993) General practitioners' acceptance of the validity of chronic fatigue syndrome as a diagnosis. *NZ Med J.* **106**: 122–4.

Epstein RM, Quill TE and McWhinney IR (1999) Somatization reconsidered: incorporating the patient's experience of illness. *Arch Intern Med.* **159**: 215–22.

Fegan KG, Behan PO and Bell EJ (1983) Myalgic encephalomyelitis – report of an epidemic. *Br J Gen Pract.* **33**: 335–7.

Fukuda K, Straus SE, Hickie I *et al.* (1994) The chronic fatigue syndrome: a comprehensive approach to its definition and study. *Ann Intern Med.* **12**: 953–9.

Gunn WJ, Connell DB and Randall B (1993) Epidemiology of chronic fatigue syndrome: the Center for Disease Control Study. *Ciba Found Symp.* **173**: 83–93.

Hartz AJ, Kuhn EM, Bentler SE, Levine PH and London R (1999) Prognostic factors for persons with idiopathic chronic fatigue. *Arch Fam Med.* **8**(6): 495–501.

Hickie I, Hadzi-Pavlovic D and Ricci C (1997) Reviving the diagnosis of neurasthenia. *Psychol Med.* **27**: 989–94.

Hickie I, Hooker AW, Hadzi-Pavlovic D *et al.* (1996) Fatigue in selected primary care settings: sociodemographic and psychiatric correlates. *Med J Aust.* **164**: 585–8.

Holmes GP, Kaplan JE, Gantz N *et al.* (1988) Chronic fatigue syndrome: a working case definition. *Ann Intern Med.* **108**: 387–9.

Ho-Yen DO and McNamara I (1991) General practitioners' experience of the chronic fatigue syndrome. *Br J Gen Pract.* **41**: 324–6.

Jason LA, Richman JA, Rademaker AW *et al.* (1999) A community-based study of chronic fatigue syndrome. *Arch Intern Med.* **159**: 2129–37.

Joyce J, Hotopf M and Wessely S (1997) The prognosis of chronic fatigue and chronic fatigue syndrome : a systematic review. *Q J Med.* **90**: 223–33.

Keighley BD and Bell EJ (1983) Sporadic myalgic encephalomyelitis in a rural practice. *J R Coll Gen Practit.* **33**: 339–41.

Komaroff AL and Buchwald DS (1998) Chronic fatigue syndrome: an update. *Ann Rev Med.* **49**: 1–13.

Lawrie SM, Manders DN, Geddes JR and Pelosi AJ (1997) A population-based incidence study of chronic fatigue. *Psychol Med.* **27**: 343–53.

Levenstein JH, McCracken EC, McWhinney IR, Stewart MA and Brown JB (1986) The patient-centered clinical method. *Fam Pract.* **3**: 24–30.

Levine PH, Snow PG, Ranum BA, Paul C and Holmes MJ (1997) Epidemic neuromyasthenia and chronic fatigue syndrome in West Otago, New Zealand: a 10-year follow-up. *Arch Intern Med.* **157**: 750–4.

Lewis G and Wessely S (1992) The epidemiology of fatigue: more questions than answers. *J Epidemiol Comm Health.* **46**: 92–7.

Lloyd AR, Hickie I, Boughton CR, Spencer O and Wakefield D (1990) Prevalence of chronic fatigue syndrome in an Australian population. *Med J Austr.* **153**: 522–8.

Lloyd AR, Wakefield D, Boughton C and Dwyer J (1988) What is myalgic encephalomyelitis? *Lancet.* **1**: 1286–7.

Marinker M (1983) Communication in general practice. In: D Pendleton and J Hasler (eds) *Doctor–Patient Communication*. Academic Press, London, UK.

McEvedy CP and Beard AW (1970) Royal Free Epidemic of 1955: a reconsideration. *BMJ*. 1: 7–11.

McIlvenny SP (1998) *Fatigue in a developing country* 'Thesis'. Queen's University, Belfast, Northern Ireland. Unpublished.

McWhinney IR (1984) Changing models: the impact of Kuhn's theory on medicine. *Fam Pract*. **1**: 3–8.

McWhinney IR (1997) *A Textbook of Family Medicine*. Oxford University Press, New York.

Murdoch JC (1987) Myalgic encephalomyelitis (ME) syndrome – an analysis of the findings in 200 cases. *N Z Fam Physician*. **14**: 51–4.

Murdoch JC (1988a) *ME Syndrome. Therapeutic notes No. 205*. Department of Health, Wellington, New Zealand.

Murdoch JC (1988b) Cell-mediated immunity in myalgic encephalomyelitis syndrome. *N Z Med J*. **101**: 511–12.

Murdoch JC (1995) *Chronic fatigue syndrome: the patient-centered view*. Paper presented at conference 'ME: the patient-oriented approach', 10–12 February, Dunedin, New Zealand.

Pawlikowska T, Chalder T, Hirsch SR *et al.* (1994) Population study of fatigue and psychological distress. *BMJ*. **308**: 763–6.

Poore M, Snow P and Paul C (1984) An unexplained illness in West Otago. *N Z Med J*. **97**: 351–4.

Royal New Zealand College of General Practitioners (1985) *A survey of general practitioners' attitudes to myalgic encephalomyelitis*. Unpublished.

Sharpe MC, Archard LC, Banatavala JE *et al.* (1991) A report: chronic fatigue syndrome: guidelines for research. *J R Soc Med*. **84**: 118–21.

Simpson LO, Murdoch JC and Herbison P (1993) Red-cell shape changes following trigger finger fatigue in subjects with chronic fatigue and healthy controls. *N Z Med J*. **106**: 104–7.

Stewart M, Brown JB, Weston WW *et al.* (1995) *Patient-Centered Medicine: transforming the clinical method*. Sage Publications, Thousand Oaks, CA.

Vercoulen JH, Swanink CM, Fennis JF *et al.* (1996) Prognosis in chronic fatigue syndrome: a prospective study on the natural course. *J Neurol Neurosurg Psychiatry*. **60**: 489–94.

Wessely S, Chalder T, Hirsch S, Wallace P and Wright D (1997) The prevalence and morbidity of chronic fatigue and chronic fatigue syndrome: a prospective primary care study. *Am J Pub Health*. **89**: 1449–55.

Wessely S, Nimnuan C and Sharpe M (1999) Functional somatic syndromes: one or many? *Lancet*. **354**(9182): 936–9.

Wilson A, Hickie I, Lloyd A *et al.* (1994) Longitudinal study of outcome of chronic fatigue syndrome. *BMJ*. **308**: 756–9.

Wood ML (1991) Naming the illness: the power of words. *Fam Med*. **23**: 534–8.

The illness experience

Case study
Every day is a nightmare for Wendy Jones. After a restless night, she wakes still suffering from extreme lethargy, muscle aches and pains and feeling very down. The happy days of her pregnancy and the birth of her second child are now a very distant memory. 'Everything' now seems to be wrong. Her eyes hurt and she can't cope with the fluorescent lights inside or the sun outside. Her ears ring. Food is no longer enjoyable and she suffers from alternate diarrhea and constipation. All her muscles ache, the skin on her body is painful and her limbs are occasionally very itchy for no apparent reason. She can't seem to 'think straight'. She had always been able to cope and it was only during the last pregnancy that she had given up paid employment. Now she feels so helpless and guilty as she phones her mother once again and asks her to come over and help with the children. She hopes Willie will not find out that Mum has been here again. When her mother comes over she wishes she hadn't bothered because she, too, is all stressed out and goes on and on about how Wendy should take her father's advice and go to LA for the new tests. Sometimes she feels tempted to end it all. The fatigue never seems to let up. She feels so terrible, it would be difficult to explain just how bad it is to others, even if her cognitive faculties could achieve that level of reflection.

She goes to see her doctor again but that is a waste of time because he is not helpful. This is a puzzle because he was a great help during her pregnancy and he delivered the baby. Now he keeps asking her how her marriage is (OK before all this), is there any stress at home (is there ever!) and is there any other stress in her life? (what a stupid question!) For some reason she is left feeling that the symptoms she has don't fit into the diagnoses he knows about, and that somehow her symptoms aren't real and the illness is her 'fault'. The doctor's cold attitude and behavior puzzle her. All these questions about waking up early when she can't get to sleep at all, and asking her if she had ever contemplated suicide (how did he know?). He had given her some pills but they had made her feel worse. She wonders whether they might help her end it all.

Documenting the testimony

One of the great difficulties that a doctor encounters in writing about the patient's experience is that the stories of sickness which he or she has heard from people are already modified by the time they are given in the consultation and even more so by the time they are interpreted. People tell us what they think we want to hear and we, the doctors, tend to water down what they say to fit what our current theories of illness are. Doctors, as we shall see later on, are the most powerful legitimizers of the sick role in modern society, and therefore are still greatly feared and protected. Few of us have the insight into the paradoxical nature of our role portrayed by writers like Salman Rushdie (Rushdie, 1983)

> What is a doctor, after all? A legitimised voyeur, a stranger whom we permit to poke fingers and even hands into places where we would not permit most people to insert so much as a finger tip; who gazes on what we take most trouble to hide; a sitter at bedsides, an outsider admitted to our most intimate moments (birth, death, etc.) anonymous, a minor character, yet paradoxically central, especially at the crisis.

At this crisis the main message is strangely minimized by one of the two players. The area of the subjective, what people feel, or say they feel, has come to assume a minor role in modern medicine and Dr Rose is not an exception to this rule. The story which I tell about my symptoms seems always less important than what a doctor or a test can demonstrate about them. The problem here is the concern within medicine for scientific proof and this path has been taken because it was successful in solving some really important medical problems.

Medicine's positivist heritage

When a 19th century person went to a doctor and said 'For the past few weeks I have felt very thirsty and I seem to be continually passing water', this personal statement of symptoms was translated into diabetes (literally in 'passing through'). In turn, this passing through was differentiated into two types by examining the urine, in the past a taste, but latterly a test. Thus, the diabetes was either sweet (mellitus) or tasteless (insipidus). Because of the apparent simplicity of this approach the convention was established that people with the same illness ought to have most things in common (abstractions) and that these ought to be able to be generalized to other people with a view to improving diagnosis. The influence of positivism, i.e. only accepting those things which can be demonstrated by scientific experiment, left us with only two forms of diabetes, mellitus and insipidus, later found to be caused by a lack of antidiuretic hormone by the hypothalamus. Of course, most cases of *tasteless passing through* had nothing whatever to do with the hypothalamus and had more to do with the enlargement of the prostate, overanxiety or the ingestion of too much water or beer. In spite of this, doctors now value the concept and the person who talks about urine passing through will almost always be tested for diabetes.

Many of the medical problems with yes/no answers can now been solved if by the verb 'solve' you mean coming to a scientific diagnosis. For example, an 18-month-old boy was diagnosed in 1999 with diabetes mellitus by his doctor, because he wondered why he was having so many infections and answered the question *Does he have diabetes mellitus?* by measuring his serum glucose. The answer to the question was *Yes* and a very important answer it was. The great value of the blood test in making this very important diagnosis reinforces the desire of doctors to find simple answers to all the problems encountered in daily practice, and this convention of dualistic thinking appears to be a convenient way of keeping the problem small enough to be handled by a busy, sometimes stressed medical practitioner. However, what is often forgotten is that the convention is made much more efficient by the free presentation of symptoms, in his case by his mother's anxiety that he did not look well and that her other children did not act like this at that age. This free presentation of symptoms is even more important when the solution is not quite as simple as looking at the throat or testing the urine, as is the case with Wendy Jones.

Medicine has developed convenient shortcuts that allow Wendy's doctor to work quickly and efficiently in his everyday practice. He has learned in medical school that certain symptoms presented by the patient usually betray the presence of certain diseases. So, passing water frequently can mean diabetes, chest pain can mean heart disease, abdominal pain can mean gastric or duodenal ulcer or appendicitis. However, the importance of these shortcuts has been greatly exaggerated. In general practice they occur in percentages large enough to keep trying but too small for maximum efficiency. When we encounter symptom complexes such as chronic fatigue or CFS, we use the shortcuts. Indeed the criteria described in Chapter 1 include such shortcuts as testing the hemoglobin or thyroid hormone which is going to be positive in less than 5% of the tests carried out.

Even where the diagnostic shortcuts result in negative answers we try the shortcut of symptomatic treatment. Like our historical forebear, the apothecary, the family doctor is often like a shopkeeper standing behind the counter, matching the customers' symptoms with the bottles of medicine behind in the treatment of presenting symptoms. The patient with multiple symptoms, in turn, can end up taking many remedies for her or his individual symptoms. While we have to agree that these shortcuts have been very useful in the solution of medical problems, medical practice has devolved into a process where we search for the gold of positive diagnoses in what we tend to regard as the dross of symptoms. We check full blood counts, erythrocyte sedimentation rates, blood pressures, serum lipids, X-rays and ultrasound scans. We poke endoscopes in even more intimate places than the finger can reach and we pride ourselves in discovering disease even before the person has been able to develop the symptoms associated with it.

Because of this development, the same pressure for a shortcut has been operating in the case of people with CFS. Much of the research which will be reported in Chapter 3 is a search for this shortcut driven largely by the potential profit engendered by doing tests in the millions who are affected. Again and again we hear people say 'If only there was a simple test for CFS, the problem would be solved'. According to this logic we would then have positive (sweet) CFS and negative (non-sweet) CFS. It cannot be denied that any advance on this front would be extremely helpful. If Wendy's CFS test were positive we could predict that Dr Rose would at least be interested in her. However, if it were negative, he would probably jump to the conclusion that CFS was a genuine disorder and as this one definitely isn't CFS her problem is just psychological, and Wendy would be no better off.

The analogy of diabetes is therefore not a very helpful one because there is no such simple shortcut in the scientific evaluation of most of our current medical problems. All diseases are multilevel disorders with complex problems involving the physical, psychological, social and spiritual levels. For thousands of years people have gone to physicians with the complaint of water passing through, and in the past the sweet taste only predicted certain death. In the 1930s the understanding of the medical profession became more adequate to the management of diabetes because these people could be identified as a distinct diagnostic group. However, the knowledge that lack of insulin was common to all diabetics did not solve all the problems of diabetes. Fear of death, fear of blindness and other complications is still a problem for the person with diabetes and their families and for the doctors who care for them. The mother of our little boy with diabetes gets depressed and worries about him. Similarly, the problems of having a baby with Down's syndrome did not disappear when it was discovered in 1959 that such children had an extra chromosome 21. It is obvious that these shortcuts of laboratory diagnosis have improved the management of the conditions to which they apply but all such diagnoses bring special problems which can only be identified by listening to the account of the individual's experience. Searching for these identifying features must remain part of the doctor's agenda but they cannot be regarded as a necessary qualification for the doctor's attention.

The major problem for Wendy and her doctor is that, in attempting to identify her problem, he discards the knowledge she brings to the consultation as being unimportant. She knows that her life has become an unbearable burden and yet he fails to be impressed by the qualitative statements that she brings. He filters through the evidence that she brings and comes up with the decision that this horrific disruption of her whole life is either nothing or a psychological disturbance. While the professional bystander might be kind enough to view that opinion as banal understatement, the involved person will view it as a monstrous lie.

The tendency to discount personal experience as unimportant is an old error as can be seen from the following quote from Montaigne in the 16th century, described in the *BMJ* (1999) under the title 'Doctor's Dilemma'.

> Like him who paints the sea, rocks and heavens, and draws the model of a ship as he sits safe at his table, but send him to sea and knows not how or where to steer, so doctors often make such a description of our maladies as the town crier does of a lost dog or donkey, of such a color, such ears, etc., but bring the very animal before him and he knows it not for all that.
> Michel de Montaigne (1533–92)

For this error we can blame the scientific training of doctors which has taught them that the only reliable knowledge is that which can be objectively evaluated. So if the patient claims to be unwell but the blood tests are normal, then the patient must be well. The patient could be a John Keats and talk about *the wakeful anguish of the soul* but that will be to no avail unless examination of his body tells a different story. This accounts for the fact that thousands of people with CFS have been told by doctors that there is *nothing wrong*. Our problem lies in our theory of knowledge and to understand illnesses such as CFS we need to expand our definition of what constitutes valid knowledge.

Expanding medicine's theory of knowledge

EF Schumacher (1977) described four fields of knowledge.

- What is going on in my own inner world?
- What is going on in the inner world of other beings?
- What do I look like in the eyes of other beings?
- What do I observe in the world around me?

It is the fourth field, constituting the area of scientific inquiry, which has been the foundation of scientific medicine and which has been responsible for many scientific advances and the resolution of individual suffering. However, it seems that scientific medicine has often limited the fourth field to what is happening in the dead body of the patient. Often other observations, such as evidence which comes from the social world or the patients' descriptions of their inner world, are dismissed as irrelevant. The doctor is supposed to be observing the world, not just a minute portion of the patient's body, and such limited observations are not truly scientific.

However, in Wendy's case, what needs to be explored is the inner world of her suffering and the only key to that world is her description of what she is going through. It may well be that, having heard the description, the doctor may discount its level of importance, maybe even label it as delusion, but the problem is that many doctors dismiss and discard the description as unimportant even before it is given or, worse still, refuse to listen at all. The effect is the same; a denial of the patient's reality.

In the unpublished study of people with CFS in New Zealand (Murdoch, 1995), virtually all first consulted their own doctor and a third rated the encounter as 'unhelpful' or 'very unhelpful'. While this outcome is better than the experience in other areas of disability – over half of the mothers of Down's syndrome babies coming home from hospital in Scotland found their doctors unhelpful (Murdoch, 1984) – it is useful to explore why these unsatisfactory communications occur. Perhaps one of the problems is a lack of shared reality. Reality has different meanings for patient and doctor and there should be no requirement to discount one's own reality in the patient–doctor interaction. However, there is a requirement to receive evidence from the other point of view.

A person like Wendy is concerned with the reality of living with her fatigue, sleep disturbance, physical pain, misery and cognitive confusion. If we examine her fields of knowledge:

- What is going on in my own inner world?
- What is going on in the inner world of other beings?
- What do I look like in the eyes of other beings?
- What do I observe in the world around me?

we will find that she is mainly in Field 1, whereas if we examine the fields of knowledge of Dr Rose, he is mainly in Field 4, but only in a very limited way. Conflict is inevitable because they miss each other's reality by a long way. Schumacher (1977) put it this way:

> When the level of the knower is not adequate to the level of the object of knowledge, the result is not a factual error, but something much more serious: an inadequate and impoverished view of reality.

So, Wendy and her doctor drift apart and the one who suffers is Wendy. However, the doctor's professional standard as a scientist also suffers because he is not making an objective analysis of the experience she brings to him. The raw material he should be working with is the experience of her illness. He must meet her on levels one and two of this exploration of her inner world if he is to help her to heal from the disruption of her life world caused by her symptoms. Neither the doctor nor the patient should seek to modify or interpret the account of these experiences before they have been given a hearing, because they constitute the main evidence on which a diagnosis is going to be made. In listening, doctors should look first to the experience of the inner world to see if the account brings echoes of recognition and compassion. The judgment can be made later but first the witness must be allowed to tell the story as it is.

This 'telling it as it really is' is a profoundly important and spiritual part of the patient–doctor consultation. The decision to impart this truly privileged information depends on how desperate is the need of the person suffering and the safety he or she feels in the presence of the person being consulted. It is as if the person takes out a piece of the finest, most fragile porcelain and hands it for safe-keeping to the doctor. It is to be handled with extreme care, admired and handed back for safe keeping to the only one who can retain it and evaluate it.

Stories of the sickness chronic fatigue syndrome

There are immense similarities in the stories of patients, and later a number of areas where similarities or disparities arise will be described.

- The problems of getting a diagnosis.
- The attitudes of health professionals to an illness that does not fit their medical models.
- The social stigma that comes from an illness that is poorly recognized and frequently overlaid with derogatory labels of the kind that suggest that the patients are choosing to be ill and it is, therefore, their fault that they are so miserable.
- Therefore, as the illness is considered to be self-generated, the patient should not need nor expect any assistance, support or resources for their recovery.

As we started to write this chapter we wanted to write about the experiences as we had been taught to write for the academic world: conceptually, with short two-to-six line quotes to illustrate the points we were trying to make. But just as CFS does not fit medicine's square of knowledge, neither does the experience of CFS fit the academic world's expectations of good work. Rather than force-fitting them into our world, relatively long quotations have been chosen as exemplars of the many available, with additional editorial comment restricted to points of clarification. Quotations have been chosen from published literature and also from previously unpublished portions of research on patient self-management in CFS undertaken by HDP. While some aspects of the research findings have been published (Denz-Penhey *et al.*, 1999), these quotes were part of the mass of data collected but not previously used in publications.

First experiences

Four years ago I was diagnosed as having chronic fatigue syndrome (CFS). Imagine for a moment that you are the subjective patient, not the objective physician. You catch 'a cold' and thereafter the quality of your life is indelibly altered. You can't think clearly ... sometimes it's all you can do to read the newspaper or to follow the plot of a television program. Jet lag without end. You inch along the fog-shrouded precipice of patient care, where once you walked with confidence. Myalgias wander about your body with no apparent pattern. Symptoms come and go, wax and wane. What is true today may be partially true tomorrow or totally false next week. You know that sounds flaky, but, dammit, it's happening to you.

You are exhausted, yet you can sleep only two or three hours a night. You were a jogger who ran three miles regularly; now a walk around the block depletes your stamina. Strenuous exercise precipitates relapses that last weeks. There is nothing in your experience in medical school, residency or practice with its grueling hours and sleep deprivation that even approaches the fatigue you feel with this illness. (English, 1991)

I live in a glass cage ... myalgic encephalitis, one of the chronic fatigue syndromes. I was a general practitioner when the first symptoms appeared three years ago, shortly after I was immunised against hepatitis B. The following month I developed glandular fever and my illness began in earnest, with multiple symptoms, which continually varied in intensity: sore throat, swollen glands, fatigue, 'brain fog', malaise, myalgia, muscle fatigue, fasciculation, sweats, postural hypotension, alcohol intolerance, poor concentration and memory, emotional lability and loss of atopic response.

Words can lie comfortably on the page, distanced by medical terminology. But this list invaded my life. Myalgia: the pain and exhaustion of the walk from my bed to the bathroom took half an hour to subside. Fatigue: my husband carried me downstairs for Sunday lunch but after one course I fell asleep, exhausted. Poor concentration: reading or watching television was often impossible. Emotional lability: at random my usual cheerful, confident self exchanged repeatedly with an unfamiliar negative, fretful character. (Fleming, 1994)

From the first 'flu' symptoms in November, 1987 until the beginning of the bizarre nightmares four months later, a constellation of symptoms emerged. They increased in number and severity each week, and occurred in a frightening, kaleidoscopic fashion; almost randomly, yet with surprising regularity. Other symptoms became permanent; photophobia, alcohol intolerance, sore throat, cystitis, regular afternoon headaches (beginning before 3 pm and refractory to almost any pain medication), heat intolerance and slow weight gain, to name many. These were accompanied by disconcerting signs: recurrent herpes simplex outbreaks, chronic tachycardia at rest, facial 'flush' from mid afternoon until bedtime, and small but palpably tender axillary lymph nodes.

Even with these symptoms and signs more bad experiences were yet to come. In April, flying an airplane by myself I twice became disoriented ... unable to understand the difference between the words left and right! Soon I was getting lost in San Jose Airport parking lot. Then attention span shrank, near-term memory went south, and word selection became an embarrassing comedy. And what did I do about all this? I went into high-gear denial, as any sensible physician would do. I was scared to death! I first laid this all to stress (as I was encouraged to do by my medical colleagues) ... Whatever it was ... I just wanted it to go away. (Harvey, 1990)

Getting a diagnosis

A thorough general medical evaluation revealed little: a few atypical lymphocytes at best. My continued dyspnea-on-exertion warranted cardiac and pulmonary function evaluations. Again, normal tests, but a provisional diagnosis of 'possible myocarditis' was made. Shortly afterward, that diagnosis, too, was ruled out following more detailed cardiac evaluation ... By now, evaluators ... were looking at me askance, mumbling 'stress'. And 'don't worry'. (Harvey, 1990)

'All the tests are normal, there's nothing wrong with you.' Well why do I feel so ill? The doctor ignored my question and changed the subject to my slightly high cholesterol levels. I asked again, what can I do about my symptoms? He smiled, shrugged his shoulders and opened the door, gently pushing me through.

Finally three doctors and several years later: 'All the tests are what I expected. From what you have told me and from my examination, you have chronic fatigue syndrome ... (brief details given) ... this is what we can do ...' Immense relief. This one believed me and now I know what's wrong. (Judy, 1993. Unpublished extract from *Self-Management Research*.)

Coping with the symptoms

I was just so tired. I can remember my two-year-old's birthday party preparations. I rang my friend and told her I had made a jelly and an instant pudding as well as tidying the house. She thought it was a joke. But I was serious. I was so proud. Normally I could never get all the house tidy at one time and anything extra at all was more than I could cope with, but I had done it. Seems amazing now I'm better, but that's the way it was.

I knew I was getting better when I could let the children bring their friends home from school. When I was bad I used to send them to other places to play. They could never bring children home. I never had the energy and I was so bad tempered. So they played away. Then I knew things were really good again when I could not only have a teenage party at home but they could stay overnight with loud music on. (Renee, 1994. Unpublished extract from *Self-Management Research*.)

Post-viral fatigue syndrome: a canker in my brain ... afternoons were a fog of frightening density. My body felt terribly heavy and when I rested on the bed I felt I had completely lost touch with it; it seemed to be unresponsive and remote. I felt nauseated by the deep fatigue and by my attempts to regain wakefulness. Now luckily I have risen above that, but other symptoms persist. The repetitive brain seems incurable and I am plagued by lapses of memory. Sections of a book read the day before are unfamiliar the next day. Books I prized highly and knew almost inside out in the past are now sketchy ghosts if remembered at all, and mostly I have no memory of them, except a faint puzzling notion that I have encountered them, like a dim recall or sensation of a forgotten dream. I meet people in the street and I realise I know them but have no idea of my connection to them. I try desperately to recall them as I make non-committal conversation. But even the conversation can seem senseless to me: for some alarming moments I think I am confronted with a foreign language ... I sit in the front room and ponder how to reach the bathroom. I have suddenly lost awareness of where it is in relation to my present position in the house ... I feel hopelessly drained by company ... Walking alone is easier than conversing with someone along the way or just coping with their presence, except that often it helps to have someone there as a kind of ballast to keep me steady. Walking can almost send me to sleep but I like to go out if I can because plenty of people cannot, and anyway I feel trapped if I stay in. (Hartnell, 1987)

When I was in my medium time, not too bad to do some things, but not good, I used to have to think about how much I could do all the time. If I went to town I would know that my limit was six things ... five was better. And that included buying the bread for lunch and meat for tea. So that meant I could only manage another three or four things. It depended on how much traffic there was, how many people were in town, how the children behaved. But it was so frustrating. I would have to be so careful to manage the stress so I could do as much as I could before my mind stopped. It would be like . . . someone would freeze frame the TV and my mind would just stop. And here I was in town with two small children tugging at my arm and I would wonder where I was and how did I get home. I had done a university degree and managed a big office and I couldn't do some of the most basic of life's essentials . . . really hard on the ego . . . smashes self-esteem. (Helen, 1994. Unpublished extract from *Self-Management Research*.)

Patient managing the doctor managing the patient

I don't waste my visits to the doctor. I can't afford to wear my doctors out or I'll lose their sympathy and they won't take me seriously any more. So I don't talk about **everything** that's wrong, only those things that they can do something about. (Sandra, 1998. Unpublished extract from *Self-Management Research*.)

He thought I abused him because I wanted to be in control of my own health. I read up what was wrong and took that to the doctor and he didn't like it. Now I have to find a new doctor. (Sandy, 1996. Unpublished extract from *Self-Management Research*.)

Societal messages

The following are a series of general messages received by members from the Self-Management Research followed by a comment from one particular member:

You don't look sick. You'll get over it. It's all in the mind/head, you want to be sick. People who get sick get better. It's not okay to be sick a long time. Must be self-inflicted. You're just wagging from work. You should be better by now. You're getting lazy. You look all right. You're looking well today. Are you **still** sick. Why aren't you better yet? You're a bit of a fraud. There's nothing wrong with you, really. Cheer up. No-one's ever died from it. You're **always** sick. You are always sleeping.

Some think it lasts only a weekend or so. Push physically to the limits. If only you did this ... I know someone who has ME but they don't need home help, why do you? You would be healthy if you ate healthy foods. Do a little more each day, you'll improve. Get more exercise. Be more sociable. Fight it, be strong.

We've done the tests, they are all normal. There is nothing more we can medically do for you. Have you any **serious** illness? (Unpublished extract of collected statements from each of the groups in the *Self-Management Research*, 1990–96)

The bloody media. They affect what people think. A few weeks back they were reporting that all you need to do was run two miles a day to get better. So I had people telling me to go running. Like the cold bath fad years ago, have a cold bath every day and you'll get better. They want the quick-fix answer just as much as the doctors do. I've had a huge expense with quick-fix ideas. I've spent a fortune on alternative practitioners and pills and stuff. They are not necessarily any better than doctors and some are charlatans. Everyone wants a quick fix. I've now become a cynic. (Sandra, 1998. Unpublished extract from *Self-Management Research*.)

Trying the 'psychological' approach

I changed track, wondering if my disease had a psychosomatic basis. So I decided to try psychotherapy and rummaged through the cupboards of my psyche. It proved to be a challenging and rewarding experience but not the answer to my predicament. (Fleming, 1994)

I realised I wasn't strong and I was going to commit suicide. I needed help and I went to psych med to be cared for. But they didn't. They just lectured me and told me I had got it all wrong. There was no emotional support or caring at all. (Three suicide attempts occurred.) (Anon, 1985. Unpublished extract from *Self-Management Research*.)

I saw a psychiatrist for months and a therapist for two years. I did what they said even when I thought it was silly, because I knew I wasn't healthy. Took their pills too. But it didn't work. I was still ill, no better, just the same mess. If the psychological approach is so good how come it doesn't work? (Chris, 1994. Unpublished extract from *Self-Management Research*.)

The effect of the stigma of the 'psychological/psychiatric' label

Defining a set of complaints as psychosomatic places the responsibility for illness on the shoulders of the patients and, consequently, increases their suffering.

> Repeated experiences of being delegitimized in one's experience of having a 'real' illness lead to suffering in the form of frustration and anger, but especially of self-doubt. Being told time and again that, as one person put it, 'you can't be experiencing what you are experiencing', eventually leads to the questioning of perception, sensation and, ultimately, one's very rationality. Many study subjects felt compelled at one time or another to entertain the possibility that they might, after all, be 'crazy', that their illness was 'all in their heads' ... Self-doubt can precede, follow, or co-occur with the often fierce resistance to psychological interpretation that has been repeatedly observed in CFS sufferers. Patients resist a psychiatric diagnosis because ... psychological disorder is stigmatized. The origins of stigma lie in the implication of responsibility in psychiatric illness and in the naturalist paradigm devaluing of afflictions of the mind as 'imaginary'. These hidden values reveal the moral dimensions of diagnosis, naturalism and the dualistic metaphysics in which both are embedded. (Ware, 1993)

> Who wants to be labeled 'unbalanced or nutty'? If you're 'nuts' either the illness is imaginary or you're 'feeble-minded' and treated like you can't think for yourself. If it's imaginary, then you are making it (the symptoms) all up ... you don't need help, that is just pandering to you and it must stop ... it just encourages you to stay sick if they help ... so you must keep working, you can't ask for help ... and people think they can be nasty to you. You just wait for their next attack. If you're feeble-minded others have to do **everything** for you – decisions that is, not the actual work. They still expect you to work. But they don't let you ... think ... that is they don't listen to you ... they don't think you have anything to contribute ... they just put you into their preconceived mould and if you don't fit they just stuff you in anyway ... and you can't complain 'cos if you do you're just ungrateful and selfish and they are just trying to help. Doctors are the worst. They just don't listen to you when they have put a psychological label on you. They just ignore the symptoms as if they don't matter any more. And I have to pay to see him and be ignored. So I don't go any more. (Judy and Clem, 1993. Unpublished extract from *Self-Management Research*.)

> Therefore it's a vicious circle. (When they don't listen to me) I get defensive and belligerent and loud, in order to be heard. (Peter, 1993. Unpublished extract from *Self-Management Research*.)

> From time to time I go psychotic, I do go psychotic and I admit that. But I still have CFS. I still have the tiredness and muscle pain and all the rest. And last week it got really bad and I went to (the doctor). But she just went on and on about my psychiatric history. And I was okay at the time, I wasn't hallucinating or anything, but she spent the whole time going on about it. When I wanted to talk about my tiredness and pain and my shaking that was driving me crazy she told me to make another appointment and come back another day. I had run out of time. (Leslie, 1994. Unpublished extract from *Self-Management Research*.)

Leslie was in tears when she reported this. Some months later she was admitted to hospital as an acute case and diagnosed as having malignant hypertension, kidney failure and an aortic aneurysm – she is now authentic. Whether she was a 'true' CFS case might be debated but she continued to have the symptoms after the other conditions were stabilized. Her periodic psychoses may well have been due to toxicity secondary to kidney failure. Leslie is a good example of the care which is needed in not dismissing symptoms as unimportant just because the person has a current diagnosis.

Message to my colleagues

> I ask for your patience. CFS is sufficient indignity by itself; do not compound it. It takes considerable time and infinite patience to take an accurate history from a frail patient with impaired memory and concentration, especially if that history is long and complex. But if you take that time, you can do a world of good. CFS may frustrate you, but it is equally fascinating and rewarding. Resist the temptation of hurried, superficial evaluation. This is no illness for cookbook doctors. It is a disease for medical intellectuals with supple and open minds. (English, 1991)

Retrieving medicine's oral tradition

The evocative and heart-rending descriptions of the suffering of people with CFS have been widely published and there is no doubt that pressure from the people and the media has led to a re-examination of the place of the subjective in the evaluation of an illness. The study of how people feel illness needs to be regarded is just as important as the search for the pathophysiological processes which underlie the illness and which may lead to specific treatments. The important issue is to recognize the footprints left in the sand by the experience and there are plenty of these footprints which indicate the condition if only we care to look. In the case of CFS we have a classification based on subjective criteria and there are many similar examples of illnesses which have no obvious abnormalities in the blood, the organs or the tissues to explain them. Others include irritable bowel syndrome, fibromyalgia syndrome and depressive illness.

In an important paper subtitled *I can't hear you while I'm listening*, Baron (1985) has emphasized the great gulf which exists between the way we think about disease as physicians and the way we experience it as people. Some of the most evocative descriptions above came from physicians who had become ill with CFS (English, 1991; Fleming, 1994; Harvey, 1990). Sometimes physicians forget that they are people, and it takes an encounter with their own symptoms to remind them of reality. However, Baron points out that the experience of illness seems to be intimately related to a sense of disorder, of loss of control, of things not being right with the world. Wendy's world is in chaos. All the things in her life she took for granted, her love for Willie, her pride in motherhood, her superwoman status have spun off out of control and out of memory. One of the tasks of the physician, Baron points out, is to deal with the disturbance in the person's ability to relate to and function in the world. Dr Rose should have been in a unique position to deal with this problem because he had the opportunity to observe all of these positive features in his previous meetings with her. Seen from this phenomenological point of view, Wendy comes to him not only as a case of CFS but of a dysfunctional body, a poorly coping mother and an unfulfilling partner. From her point of view her body isn't working properly, her mind isn't working properly; consequently she cannot fulfill her chosen roles and she feels miserable.

The answer, according to Baron, is to study the discipline of medical phenomenology and look at the illness from the patient's perspective but perhaps a simpler approach might be to encourage the human being in us to develop, and to reawaken the power of the oral tradition in our practice. The rich stories told us by the Wendys of this world have been minimized by our dominant visual technologies. As McWhinney (1983) has said:

> Even in writing down the patients' complaints in our own language we lose much of the richness of the original oral communication.

There is a healing role in being there and listening, of bearing witness to the statement of disorder, of saying gentle and encouraging things like 'If that had been me, I don't know how I would have coped', or, 'This is not like the Wendy

I know!' The use of such language can produce magic moments that build bridges from the past into the future. The attitude that assists this position is that of the 'insider' described by Gething (1992) in the field of disabilities. Insiders are those who have experienced regular close contact with those who are disabled and who hold a coping framework which recognizes the disability as only one aspect of a multifaceted life that includes gratifications as well as grievances, abilities as well as disabilities. In contrast, outsiders are those who have not experienced regular close contact and tend to hold negative or stereotyped views that focus on the handicap and tragedy associated with disability. Outsiders are more likely to hold a succumbing framework in which difficulties are highlighted. Emphasis is on what the person can't do, what is denied the person, the problems that weigh the person down. Such succumbing frameworks produce such terms as the 'heartsink' patient (O'Dowd, 1988). The problem with Dr Rose was that he was an outsider with respect to the problems which Wendy had. Like it or not, he has to be an insider in order to help her in this situation and his major contribution as an insider would have been to remind her of what she used to be like and how impressive she was formerly, at the same time as finding out what has caused the problem and how to help her back.

The need for matching models

Given the obvious inadequacies between the levels of the knower (the doctor) and the object of knowledge (the person with CFS) revealed by these stories, there are surely some practical lessons to be learned. The first is the necessity for doctors to check that they and the patient are actually hearing the same story. It seems incredible that two human beings can be alone in the same room and the one can be so distressed and the other so unmoved. A bridge is a structure that has firm foundations on both sides of the problem. Denial that there is a problem is a bridge to and from nowhere.

Having agreed on the same story we also have to be sure that both doctors and patients are either using the same model of illness, or understand that they are using differing models. Klasen and Goodman (2000) have demonstrated the mismatch of the explanatory models on hyperactivity held by general practitioners in the UK and the parents of children with the illness. This qualitative study demonstrated that parents and physicians saw the illness from different perspectives. Parents saw hyperactivity as a long lasting, biologically based problem that needed treatment in its own right and that benefited from diagnosis. Most of the physicians were unsure whether hyperactivity was a medical disorder warranting a label and specific treatment, and often saw it as a passing phase related to family stresses. As we shall see in the next chapter, there are several explanatory models for CFS and the same conflict will inevitably arise between most physicians and most patients.

Finally it has to be realized that *hearing* and *listening* as described by Baron (1985) are quite separate but equally important activities. According to Baron *hearing* was directed at appreciating the illness experience as described by the patient while *listening* was the collection of evidence from the patient by history, examination and investigation in order to make a differential diagnosis. The words 'hearing' and 'listening' are sometimes interchangeable, e.g. Rogers used the term 'attentive listening' to refer to the activity described as 'hearing' by Baron. The important distinction lies between the words (listening) and the meaning which the words convey (hearing). The patient-centered clinical method (Stewart *et al.*, 1995) demands the weaving back and forth between these two activities in order to reach an integrated understanding of the person's illness. The reason that this doctor can ignore the crisis, the crash and the drama is that he cannot do both activities at once and therefore his only course of action is to concentrate on listening and to refuse to hear what she is trying to tell him about her ideas, expectations and feelings about what is happening to her. Unhindered by her evidence he can decide that she does not have a crisis, a crash or a drama. Wendy's illness is classified as a minor psychiatric disorder that will be solved by six weeks on antidepressants and 'sorting herself out'. He believes he has the right or the duty, even the responsibility to ignore her reality in the light of his superior knowledge that says she does not know what she is experiencing.

The doctor who can't hear while he is listening is still around, according to the testimony of many witnesses, and he or she is as dangerous as the doctor who will do external cardiac massage but not mouth-to-mouth resuscitation. This is not an either–or situation, it has to be both. As an old Scottish politician once remarked:

> If you can't ride two horses at once, you shouldn't be in the circus.

Dr Alan Rose may be well respected by his colleagues and his patients who have something wrong with them that he recognizes but he has failed in his duty towards this patient. He has also failed to live up to the aspirations of general practice or family medicine which is different, according to McWhinney (1996) because it is a discipline which defines itself in terms or relationships, especially the patient–doctor relationship.

> Other fields define themselves in terms of content: diseases, organ systems or technologies. Clinicians in other fields form relationships with patients, but in general practice, the relationship is usually prior to content. We know people before we know what their illnesses will be.

Dr Alan Rose knew Wendy before CFS appeared, but his relationship was conditional on content. He was not a family physician but a specialist in everything that can be proved. His position denied a central value in family medicine (Marinker, 1987) which is *the uniqueness of the doctor and the patient.* This failure to value the experience of the patient was a disaster to Wendy in the short term, and in the longer term will be a disaster to both him and his espoused discipline of general practice. As Marinker has emphasized:

> If we fail to value the uniqueness of the doctor and the patient, the role of feelings and situations in the interpretation of symptoms and findings, we are condemned to be second-rate players in a second-hand game.

Conclusion

In this chapter we have attempted to describe through case records of people seen, unpublished studies, media reports and the scientific literature an identikit picture of what people with this illness experience. What we wish to emphasize is:

- the multiplicity of the symptoms
- the ferocity of their impact
- the suddenness of their onset in most populations and individuals
- the patient perspective of the search for a diagnosis
- the desperation of not being offered symptom relief without a prior diagnosis
- the isolation which comes from not being believed
- the helplessness of being put in a diagnostic box without consent.

Perhaps the lessons learned from immediate care can again be valuable in avoiding an almost inevitable conflict. Her cries for help from within the wreckage of her body and her family went unanswered. This was a case for the firemen to go in and release her, Willie and the children from the inevitable results of a terrible illness. But Dr Rose could not hear; he was only listening.

References

Baron RJ (1985) An introduction to medical phenomenology: I can't hear you while I'm listening. *Ann Intern Med.* **103**: 606–11.

De Montaigne M (1999) Doctor's dilemma. *BMJ.* **319**: 448.

Denz-Penhey H, Tilyard M, Shaw R and Harvey R (1999) Patient self-management in chronic fatigue syndrome: an action research study. *NZ Fam Physician.* **26**(1): 43–50.

English TL (1991) A piece of my mind: skeptical of skeptics. *JAMA.* **265**(8): 964.

Fleming C (1994) Personal view: the glass cage. *BMJ.* **308**: 797.

Gething L (1992) *Person to Person: a guide for professionals working with people with disabilities.* Maclennan & Petty, Sydney, Australia.

Hartnell L (1987) Post-viral fatigue syndrome: a canker in my brain. *Lancet.* **1**: 910.

Harvey WT (1990) Nightmare, neurosis, or new disease? *San Anton Med.* **43**: 21.

Klasen H and Goodman R (2000) Parents and GPs at cross-purposes over hyperactivity: a qualitative study of possible barriers to treatment. *Br J Gen Pract.* **50**: 199–202.

Marinker M (1987) Journey to the interior: the search for academic general practice. *J R Coll Gen Pract.* **37**: 385–9.

McWhinney IR (1983) Changing models: the impact of Kuhn's theory on medicine. *Fam Pract.* **1**: 3–8.

McWhinney IR (1996) The importance of being different. *Br J Gen Pract.* **146**: 433–6.

Murdoch JC (1984) Experience of mothers of Down's syndrome and spina bifida children on going home from hospital in Scotland 1971–81. *J Ment Def Res.* **28**: 123–7.

Murdoch JC (1995) Chronic fatigue syndrome: the patient-centered view. Paper presented at conference 'ME: the patient-oriented approach' 10–12 February, Dunedin, New Zealand.

O'Dowd TC (1988) Five years of heartsink patients in general practice. *BMJ.* **297**: 528–30.

Rushdie S (1983) *Shame.* Jonathan Cape, London, UK.

Schumacher EF (1977) *A Guide for the Perplexed.* Harper & Row, New York.

Stewart M, Brown JB, Weston WW *et al.* (1995) *Patient-Centered Medicine: transforming the clinical method.* Sage Publications, Thousand Oaks, CA.

Ware NC (1993) Society, mind and body in chronic fatigue syndrome: an anthropological view. *Ciba Found Symp.* **173**: 62–82.

Is there a disease called chronic fatigue syndrome?

The search for the pathophysiology of chronic fatigue syndrome

Case study
Dr Alan Rose is very puzzled by Wendy Jones, who, up to now, had been a normal, healthy person. She had occasional previous bouts of influenza, colds or other mild infections but these had been within 'normal' range of experience and had resolved in the usual timeframes. The only other times the GP had seen his patient had been during her two pregnancies, to prescribe the contraceptive pill and on one occasion for innoculations before a trip overseas. She came from a 'good' family and Alan knew her parents socially because her father was a member of the Rotary Club. Now she came with all these bizarre symptoms.

At first he thought she might be developing multiple sclerosis because of the fatigue and paresthesia but neurological examination was normal. So were all the blood tests, full blood count, erythrocyte sedimentation rate, urea and electrolytes. There was no sign of endocrine problems or indeed anything else, yet she persisted in telling him about all these symptoms. On one of her visits she had asked 'Is it ME (myalgic encephalomyelitis), doctor?' and he had been tempted to reply 'Yes, it is you' but had resisted the remark. He knew about CFS through highly emotive media coverage. He thought 'Piece of nonsense really. Why can't people like her accept that this was depression, probably a late and atypical post-natal depression', even though he had done a General Health Questionnaire (GHQ) and she was well within the normal range. He had given her some antidepressants and he hoped she would come back in two weeks feeling a little better. If not, then he would send her to the psychiatrist; in fact, she might need acute admission. All his life he had insisted on very high standards of evidence-based scientific medicine in his practice and he was not going to change that now for the sake of 'nutters' like this who were trying to prove that they had a real disease.

In this chapter we ask a very important question which arises directly from this account of Dr Alan Rose's management of Wendy. He obviously has a real problem in that he cannot recognize any familiar disease process in his patient, apart from psychiatric disorder. The problem is that he, like many doctors, has been trained using a selective biomedical and scientific model, where the patients' illness has to be explained in terms of abnormal structure and function of tissues or organs. The question is whether CFS, as defined in Chapter 1, could ever be explained in a way that would allow him and the other members of the medical profession to accept CFS as a valid illness. In many ways this has been the purpose of the research carried out into CFS over the past 60 years: to prove that it is a disease which should be included in the list of conditions that doctors such as Dr Rose are expected to identify and treat. In this chapter we will trace the process by which doctors and patients have sought to authenticate the symptom complex into a disease of proven causation. First the issue of professional power in diagnosis is addressed followed by the place of scientific evidence in making diagnoses, by looking at the descriptions of outbreaks of similar symptoms over the past 60 years to see if there is a common theme running through them. Then we will look at the abstractions which have been drawn from the various reports, e.g. atypical poliomyelitis, mass hysteria, immune dysfunction, retroviral infection, somatization disorder and note the tendency to generalize about the corporate behavior of the people with CFS on the basis of the preconceptions of the researchers. We will also discuss whether the unsuccessful attempts to explain the cause of all such illnesses under a common heading is exacerbating the problem. Finally, we will explore other ways of explaining the phenomenon and ask whether a long-term lack of an explanatory cause need necessarily preclude healing management.

Professional power

Dr Alan Rose would be horrified if we accused him of abuse of power by refusing to diagnose Wendy as having CFS but, in fact, he holds all the cards in the diagnosis as can be seen by his approach. In this court of diagnosis he is the judge, jury and executioner. He asks questions, examines her physically, orders tests and then he gives his judgment as to whether he will award her 'the sick role' or not. In this case he is prepared only to allow one possibility which is that she is depressed. To move him from this position would take a lot of persuasion. In common with most of his colleagues, he holds to an entrenched view of the world in which he works, which he acquired at the time of his undergraduate medical education and has been reinforced during his 20 years of practice. His view is that when his patients (and he really does believe that they are his) come to him for advice it is his duty to give an honest diagnosis, prognosis and valid treatment which has been proven from a scientific point of view. Thomas Kuhn (1967) called this set of received beliefs a paradigm and Dr Rose acquired these mainly during his time when he did his premedical science degree in the 1960s. Whether the people back at his old college still hold that paradigm he would have no idea. He works on his own most of the time and very rarely discusses this or any world view with anyone, but if pressed he would probably claim that he adopts it because he has confidence in what 'science' has provided to humanity in the shape of real progress. He can now prescribe antibiotics for infections, he can prevent infections through immunization, he can order tests that will reliably diagnose cancer, he can operate guidelines that will manage a whole host of common and rare diseases. In fact he, his patients and his colleagues agree that he is a very good doctor although some of his patients, including Wendy, might introduce the proviso 'provided you've got something wrong with you that he recognizes and understands'. How often that happens is a good question that the Dr Roses of this world won't discuss.

However, others who, like him, work in general practice have looked at the problem and have come up with some specific but startling answers. McWhinney (1984) has estimated from various studies that only between 21% and 50% of patients presenting in primary care with common complaints (e.g. chest pain, abdominal pain and headache) receive a specific diagnosis (e.g. heart attack, appendicitis and migraine). So most of the time, Dr Rose has really no idea of the diagnosis in his patients. How does he deal with that problem? He does this by an unquestioning belief in a concept called positivism that, simply stated, means he holds a philosophy that recognizes only these things for which he has proof. Of course, this approach does not actually help address the common complaints presented to him and we suspect that Dr Rose would treat any patient who came back time and again with unexplained chest pain or abdominal pain or headaches in the same way as he treated Wendy. A more accurate view would be that like many doctors he avoids any position that might not satisfy his selective demands. This is a doctor-centered rather than a scientific approach for he does not require proof of his belief that the 'story' that he makes up about Wendy's illness can be proven to cause the symptoms. He cannot feel Wendy's symptoms, he cannot measure her fatigue and he cannot find any change in her blood tests. Therefore, she is well and healthy according to this concept. He is like a man who has lost his car keys in the dark, but will only look for them under the street lamp even though he knows that he dropped them elsewhere. This for him is the safe approach, using only a few well-documented and proven diagnoses in his list of possibilities for Wendy.

Of course it worries him when he meets someone like this who seems to have a lot of complaints but has few measurable signs to show for it. However, he has read quite a lot about this and if the tests are all normal and the patient continues to complain, then it is obvious that they have a somatoform disorder. Somatization is

> a tendency to experience and communicate somatic distress and symptoms unaccounted for by pathological findings, to attribute them to physical illness, and to seek medical help for them. (Lipowski, 1988)

From his reading in psychiatry, he has a very good explanation for Wendy's symptoms which is that she has various conflicts in her life, e.g. Willie's being laid off, the conflict between him and her parents, the two young children, the recent pregnancy. She obviously cannot face these conflicts and her symptoms are a defence mechanism by which she can avoid dealing with the conflict and gain some relief from her threatening circumstances. Of course there is no scientific proof for this story, just as there is no diagnostic test for the label of depression which he would really prefer to give her. Unfortunately, however, he asked her the questions in the General Health Questionnaire and she did not get enough points to be labeled as having depression. Such a diagnosis would have over-ruled his original one of somatization disorder. He does not like giving her the label of somatization disorder, because she comes from a good family and has been a good patient who always seemed to accept his diagnoses. However, it would be intolerable for him not to be able to diagnose her and the term 'somatization disorder' seems appropriate. He feels unable to discuss all this with Wendy as he finds such patients are often offended by being labeled in this way. He does not recognize that he swings alternately between his dual diagnoses of somatization and atypical depression. He would like to refer her and she will soon hear the words heard by almost every severely fatigued patient, 'Have you ever thought of seeing a psychiatrist?'

Science and medicine

What we have to ask is whether these assumptions of Dr Rose's are really scientific. If he were a laboratory scientist where his 'patients' were little rats running about in cages, or chemicals being mixed in a test tube, surely the key to his experiments would be the observation of the behavior of his laboratory animals or chemicals. If laboratory animals are obviously 'ill' the scientists do not make up a bizarre story about 'psychological conflict' being the cause. They go looking for a physical cause, just like doctors do. Similarly, chemicals that don't react as expected would not be explained by a 'conflict' type justification. Any scientist would be laughed out of the lab.

So what is science in this setting? Engel (1988) quotes the definition of Odegaard thus:

> Science represents man's most persistent effort to extend and organize knowledge by reasoned efforts that ultimately depend on evidence that can be consensually validated.

In the light of that definition, Dr Rose's approach is unscientific because the object of the study is Wendy's problem and he is manifestly not extending and organizing knowledge about that problem by collecting relevant evidence. Neither is he attempting any validation with the consent of the observer of the evidence; Wendy herself. There are ways of understanding the problem of CFS from a scientific point of view. What Dr Rose does not understand is that he can still be scientific and extend and organize his knowledge of what is going on in Wendy's life. It is this organized curiosity as opposed to sterile exclusion that marks the modern physician who makes a scientific study of such illnesses.

The beginning of this task is the description of the problem. In his essay on Science and Literature, Sir Peter Medawar (1984) observed that:

> In classical inductive theories of scientific method, plain factual truth is what scientific reasoning is supposed to begin with. We start with an exact apprehension of the facts of the case, with a reliable transcript of the evidences of the senses which inductive reasoning can thereupon compound into more general truths or natural laws ... Scientific theories begin as imaginative constructions. They begin, if you like, as stories, and the purpose of the critical or rectifying episode in scientific reasoning is precisely to find out whether or not these stories are stories about real life.

The physician in clinical practice is well placed to produce these reliable transcripts but it is important that the prejudices of those who carry out the research do not interfere with the evidence of their senses. Much of modern medical practice is about trying to match the symptoms of patients with a diagnosis, but, as we have seen, this is successful in only a minority of cases. The production of a checklist of diseases whose cause is known and whose treatment is proven is one valid aspect of research, but there are other outcomes such as the identification of clinical situations where the cause is unknown or multiple. In order to do this, we have to see each patient and her or his symptoms as a new challenge to be understood by the process of clinical research. The methods we use in such research need to be appropriate to the clinical situation and we cannot limit research to the methods that are successful in the laboratory or the post-mortem room.

Feinstein (1970) has argued that any basic science for clinical medicine must include information about how to make both explanatory and managerial decisions.

The practice of clinical medicine involves two different types of decisions about the phenomena that doctors observe in their patients. In a series of explanatory decisions, doctors give names to the observed phenomena, and provide concepts to account for the causes and mechanisms that presumably created the phenomena. In a series of managerial decisions, doctors choose strategies of intervention to prevent the phenomena from occurring or to alter them after they have occurred. The explanatory decisions lead to intellectual conclusions about ideas such as diagnosis and pathogenesis of disease; the managerial decisions lead to therapeutic actions, in which the patient is treated to thwart what might happen or remedy what has occurred.

To these two aspects must be added the fact that the clinical encounter between the doctor and the patient is constantly changing both. In the history of the research into CFS described below, researchers have been accused of having become the victim of altered medical perception as if allowing any evidence from the patient to change your views were a scientific error. This is evidence of an old-fashioned world view which continues to dominate medicine (Engel, 1988). The 17th century scientist believed he could be totally objective in studying his subject, while the 21st century scientist knows that this is impossible and that she or he has to come up with better ways of understanding what is going on.

The physician who meets with Wendy must give priority to the managerial decisions such as how her distress is going to be handled so that she can give maximal care to her children, and what name will be given to the illness so that her husband and parents feel comfortable in helping her. It is important to stress that these are valid subjects for scientific inquiry. Feinstein concluded that the challenges of this new basic science of what he called clinical management included reducing observer variation, developing new systems of taxonomy, establishing criteria for diverse clinical judgments and improving qualification for 'normality', prognosis and therapy. All of these advances have to be made by those who attempt to make a scientific study of CFS.

Plain facts to general truths

So what is the result of the research produced in the case of CFS? Has the scientific community succeeded in producing general truths from the plain facts surrounding the outbreaks of fatiguing illness which have been described? The bulk of the evidence produced has been relatively recent. In the period 1966–74 there were only 1.6 citations per year in the international medical research literature (Medline) using the headings of Chronic Fatigue Syndrome, Chronic Fatigue and Immunodeficiency Syndrome and Myalgic Encephalomyelitis; in the period 1993–98 there were 183 citations per year, an increase of 11 437.5% (183/1.6). In February 2000 there were a total of 1846 citations on CFS in *Index Medicus*.

However, there is now background literature produced over the past 50 to 60 years in which doctors and scientists from a variety of backgrounds have reported the symptoms which people developed, the results of investigations and then have gone on to discuss the possible explanations as to why they should have become ill in that way. In summarizing that research we have used an important qualification for inclusion drawn from Medawar's definition. We have included accounts and research findings which have come from those who have made factual observations and not included those who try to match reports of CFS with their own theories.

The struggle to be serious about the scientific study of this illness has been strengthened by taking place against a background where many people have been openly disdainful about those who dare to have such symptoms and those researchers who take them seriously. The normally fair columns of the medical journals have been reduced to the level of farce by the publication of theories that openly deride the person with unexplained symptoms. Historians such as Shorter (1992) claim that such poor creatures are the 20th century equivalents of 19th century people with hysterical paralysis. His generalizations include:

> A whole subculture of chronic fatigue has arisen in which those patients too tired to walk give each other hints about how to handle a wheelchair and exchange notes about how to secure disability payments from the government or from insurance companies. The whirl of activities within this subculture sounds so diverting that one can understand why members would be reluctant to part with their symptoms.

Another example was provided by Richmond published under the amusing (except to sufferers) title of 'Myalgic encephalomyelitis, Princess Aurora and the wandering womb' by the *BMJ* (1989). In it she describes ME, now known as CFS, as:

> a new name for an old disease with an impressive history of synonyms. It's a British disease, unknown in the New World: but North America is in the grip of chronic Epstein–Barr virus infection, and Australasia has repetitive strain injury, which unkind people say is myalgic compensationitis.

There is no link in any of this with factual observations in people with the problem. However, the fact that they are so quickly published and so eagerly received by doctors indicates the authoritarian bias of the profession. Shorter links the epidemic of chronic fatigue to the increasing power of the media and the loss of medical authority but concedes that it is not the role of the historian to determine whether the current epidemic of CFS is *the result of epidemically spreading organic disease or of a psychic epidemic.*

The early literature

In 1959 Dr ED Acheson, later the Chief Medical Officer of England and Wales, summarized the accounts of 14 outbreaks which had occurred up to that date in such geographically differing locations as Iceland, Australia, Alaska, South Africa and various parts of the US and Europe. Half of these were doctors and nurses in hospitals and nursing homes and one outbreak was at the Royal Free Hospital in London. The claim by Acheson that these should be regarded as the same disease was based on a common clinical pattern and the characteristic sequelae.

The typical clinical features that all 14 outbreaks had in common according to Acheson were:

- headache
- myalgia or painful muscles
- paresis or paralysis
- symptoms and signs suggesting damage to the central nervous system (CNS)
- mental symptoms
- low or absent fever in most cases
- no mortality.

Other features were:

- a higher frequency in women
- a predominantly normal cerebrospinal fluid, and
- relapses which have occurred in almost every outbreak.

Only two of these would now give us significant problems and these are the presence of paresis and paralysis, and damage to the CNS. Given that the great fear in all these outbreaks was that the patients were developing poliomyelitis, it is perhaps not surprising that these were reported. Perhaps the trigger in these cases was the poliomyelitis virus causing the high prevalence of paralysis in the early stages but there is also some suggestion that full neurological examinations were not always carried out and perhaps the fear of what might happen caused the physicians to record more abnormalities than were really present. Reading through the accounts of 40 years ago it is easy to recognize the same features as have been present in Wendy and the many thousands of people who have had the illness throughout the world ever since. It is unfortunate that it took such a long time for these criteria to be agreed but the fact is that most of the arguments took place over what might be the possible cause of the problem.

The first-reported outbreak of the illness generally accepted to be CFS came in the description of an atypical form of polio affecting mainly nurses in the midst of the 1934 Los Angeles poliomyelitis epidemic. This was followed by descriptions of outbreaks in Akureyri in Iceland (1948), Adelaide in Australia (1949), New York State (1950), Coventry (1953) and the Middlesex Hospital (1952). In all the cases reviewed by Acheson it was thought that the polio virus might be involved but no evidence was found of it or other viruses in the investigations. In the research currency of the time, such negative results were enough to allow most physicians to ignore the problem. Doctors were used to seeing the obvious results of the destruction of the nervous system by the polio virus and it was very difficult for them to be impressed by such 'functional' symptoms as fatigue, memory loss and sleep disorders. Anyway, nobody seemed to die and most of the people affected seemed to be women. The matter was left to be pursued by a few zealot doctors who were convinced that there was a genuine disease, and by the minority of patients who had to face recurring symptoms long after the original outbreak.

The great unwritten theme underlying many of these early outbreaks arose from the fact that many of those affected were doctors and nurses working in hospitals or other institutions. All the medical writers of these days, including Acheson, were careful to follow the rules of the day and to write in a very objective fashion. Few of the descriptions contained any personal account of what it felt like to be ill, but the fact that doctors were ill themselves, well-hidden out of concern that bias might be claimed to be present, was undoubtedly the driving force behind the desire to see these illnesses as one clinical entity and to find a common cause. The Royal Free Hospital outbreak (1957) affected 292 of the 2500 people on the hospital staff. 18.6% of the nurses and 13.5% of the medical staff were affected and so there must have been many doctors who had the illness. The passion with which a possible cause was pursued by these doctors indicates that they wished to tell the story of the persons affected by the illness but in those days it was not considered correct to betray any personal bias and so no hint was given in the literature.

Equally, there were those who wished to debunk the whole claim that CFS was 'a real illness'. This lobby seemed to triumph in 1970 when two papers were published (McEvedy and Beard, 1970a, b) analysing the Royal Free and other outbreaks and dismissing all the cases reported by Acheson as being explained by one of two factors; mass hysteria and altered medical perception.

These papers were remarkable in that they were accepted by the *BMJ* even though they contained no original research but were merely a review of data already published 10–15 years before. If they had been papers on microbiology they would never have been published because they presented no scientific evidence but were merely the opinion of two physicians.

The theory of mass hysteria fitted well with the fact that the outbreaks of illness had happened mainly in institutions. It also suited a doctor-centered view that patients saw illness as a desirable state and that doctors should be careful in deciding who may or may not be given the societal support to do so. An editorial (1970) accompanying McEvedy and Beard's papers in the *BMJ* entitled 'Epidemic Malaise' opened with the statement that:

> The epidemic spread of panic-stricken, fanatical and hysterical behaviour, the so-called madness of crowds, was commonplace until a few centuries ago ... Affected communities tend to be relatively isolated and are often marked by a cohesion that springs from common purposes or shared emotions.

It then demonstrated a strongly negative gender bias by saying that:

> The epidemic spread of panic-stricken and hysterical conduct has been more characteristic of women.

The editorial does, however, contain a very precise description of the major symptoms of CFS:

> There was intense malaise and symptoms such as headache, sore throat, lassitude, dizziness, stiff neck, pains in limbs and back, and hyperventilation with tetanic spasms were relatively common. Pyrexia was slight or absent. Motor weakness was common but objective neurological signs were in most cases absent.

However, the importance of the symptoms was denied by the extraordinary illusion that because women were the primary sufferers, the symptoms could then be ignored. This prejudice is well illustrated by such statements as:

> Patients, male members of staff and other members of the community appeared to be notably immune to the presumed infection.

The fact that 13.5% of medical staff (virtually all male at that date) in the Royal Free outbreak also were affected was conveniently ignored.

The tradition in scientific journals of the time was to publish unsigned editorials in the same journal as important scientific papers. These editorials were intended to summarize the research so far on the topic and to draw scientific generalizations. The editorial congratulated the authors for:

> performing a valuable service in drawing attention to the possible psychological origins of some outbreaks of illness that are disseminated in an explosive manner and for which a physical explanation is apt to be readily assumed. (Editorial: Epidemic Malaise, 1970)

The writer then summarized CFS to that point by saying that:

> Communities of young women living in relative seclusion appear to be particularly susceptible, but meeting with other people may lead to a fresh crop of cases and cause the spread and recrudescence of the disorder. In some epidemics the infection appears to have spread in a striking manner by physical contagion. Dramatic public announcements detailing the features of the illness will often initiate fresh outbreaks, even in places far removed from the parent epidemic ... patients who show consistent dramatic or bizarre symptoms should be separated from other members of the group.

Thus the writer summarized 30 years of reliable transcripts using the opinions of McEvedy and Beard who had never seen any of the patients involved. These two psychiatrists made their assumptions about its etiology on the basis of their own experience with respect to hysterical groups of teenagers. Just like the infectious-disease physicians before them, they probably jumped the gun on their theories concerning etiology. It would be intriguing to know what part personal prejudices played in the background in addition to mysogenist attitudes. Certainly feelings ran high between the two camps. Ramsay (1978) summed up the position of the protagonists when he stated:

> Ours is a most remarkable profession in that we pride ourselves in being highly critical and yet one of the most astounding things to me is that the profession as a whole seems to swallow a hypothesis of mass hysteria hook, line and sinker.

A further result of the McEvedy and Beard papers and accompanying editorial was an attempt to close any further scientific study of the outbreaks. In a paper describing an outbreak in a girls' school in England (May *et al.*, 1980) in which the personality of the girls affected had been studied, there appeared a remarkable recommendation:

> Whether future outbreaks of this sort should be rigorously investigated is debatable, since the investigation itself may increase the severity of the symptoms and signs.

However, the days of confined outbreaks in closed communities seemed to be over and the next phase of the phenomenon was about to occur which seemed to contradict the generalizations so eagerly accepted by the medical profession.

It is difficult to escape the conclusion that the real battle here was the defence of medical authority against the rights of persons to say that they had a real illness. A patient could have symptoms but only a doctor had the power to say what the diagnosis was. The arrogance of this position is made clear by the statements of doctors who warned that a market for somatic labels existed in the large pool of stressed-out or somaticizing patients who sought to disguise an emotional complaint or upgrade their diagnosis from a nebulous one to a legitimate disease (Shorter, 1992). Shorter was probably right when he claimed that this loss of medical authority coincided with the power of the media and the vulnerability of the lay public to fixed ideas about illness but the profession was hoisted by its own petard because these two things had been the means it had used to protect its authority.

The problem becomes community-based

In the late 1970s and 1980s a great sea change occurred in the research into CFS. Before this time the illness seemed to occur in outbreaks in closed communities such as hospitals, schools, convents, even prisons. After about 1979, the problem became increasingly recognized by doctors working in the wider community. In the UK, New Zealand, Australia and North America, physicians in primary care and internal medicine were being consulted by a large number of people who were living at home but who had the features now agreed to be the criteria for the syndrome. So in the years 1980–86, general practitioners and internists such as Ken Fagan, Brian Keighley and Brian Calder in the West of Scotland, Peter Snow and Campbell Murdoch in Otago, New Zealand and in North America were in the process of preparing reliable transcripts of evidence presented to them by people consulting them, and mobilizing sympathetic specialist colleagues such as neurologists, virologists and other scientists to help with the clarification of what all this meant in scientific terms.

Person-centered research

It is said that researchers have to be objective and that those who become involved personally with people who suffer are subject to considerable bias. This is a perversion of the truth similar to that perpetrated by those who believe that physicians should be cold, impersonal and uninvolved in the consultation. Good research is driven by curiosity and experience and the curious physician is a passionate person who asks questions as he or she meets patients, lots of patients.

Dr James Mackenzie who went into practice in Burnley in 1879 became known as 'the father of cardiology' for his painstaking research into the 'affections of the heart'. He was faced with startling new phenomena in this practice that he could not understand, such as why many pregnant women became suddenly breathless. His response (Mackenzie, 1919) was as follows.

> I studied the circulatory condition of women before pregnancy, watched them during the time they were pregnant, observed them closely during labour and the puerperium and for months and years after, I studied not only cases with damaged hearts but also many healthy women.

After doing all this, he found that he had many questions for which there no answers. Writing in 1919, Sir James reflects:

> I could not answer these questions. I turned to my textbooks for help, I ransacked libraries without avail, till at last it dawned on me that the knowledge I wanted did not exist.

There are many parallels between the search for the pathophysiology of atrial fibrillation and heart failure in the 1890s and the search for the pathophysiological basis of CFS in the 1990s.

> Having had the lack of knowledge forced upon me in this way, I wondered if I could not do something to shed light on this matter. When I started in a somewhat hesitating fashion on this quest I had no idea where it would lead me. Not only did it bring to light many new facts, but it brought to me a consciousness of the deficiency in our knowledge in fields essential to the progress of medicine, and a knowledge of methods by which some of these deficiencies could be made good.

Mackenzie's puzzles (Murdoch, 1997) were produced and his solutions were driven by the necessity to understand the people who sat in front of him in the consultation. Likewise the research questions about CFS must come from the people who consult physicians with this problem. The field of research into CFS has become dominated by researchers who, judging by their statements, seldom see a person suffering from these symptoms. Mackenzie said:

> As disease can be recognised in the living only by the symptoms it produces, a knowledge of symptoms should be an essential qualification for the investigator to possess.

This knowledge of symptoms was the contribution of those curious physicians who were largely from the same background as Dr Alan Rose but had the advantage that they were seeing many more patients with the problem. Their priority was to describe the clinical features, the criteria that have become accepted as described in Chapter 1. However, in their haste to make sense of what they were seeing in their patients, most of them adopted a research approach that was almost destined to fail: the assumption that prepacked answers would explain the phenomena being experienced by the patients. In almost every case the clinicians would link up with laboratory-based researchers and the approach would be to apply tests done in other clinical areas to see whether a conventional answer existed. This approach to research was traditional and very simple, and in some ways mirrored the clinical approach of doing a series of blood tests. It consisted in asking whether all the people studied had factors in common in the areas of virology, immunology, endocrinology and psychiatry. Given the pressure to come up with rapid answers to a difficult public health problem it was possibly a reasonable approach but the risk was, just like with the individual patient, that when none of the answers was positive we had a problem. Where could we go after we had drawn a series of blanks?

What was needed was a good question, specific to the problems posed by people like Wendy. Questions like ' What could it be that could attack previously healthy people suddenly, leave them with these symptoms for up to two years or more, and disable them so severely?' Howie (1991) has said that research questions should be important, interesting and answerable. Experience in CFS has shown that the problem lies in the third of these. As we have seen in Chapter 1, we should have spent a lot more time defining what we regarded as a case of CFS before applying the answering machine of laboratory research to the problem. We will now summarize the disappointing results of the search for an easy prepacked answer to the problem of CFS.

The continuing search for a viral cause

Most of the early research was carried out to demonstrate that CFS was an atypical form of polio and that a virus such as poliovirus was the infective agent. In later years interest shifted to Epstein–Barr and Coxsackie virus and finally to the search for the human immunodeficiency virus (HIV).

'I am sure it's some kind of virus' is the favorite statement of many doctors and patients searching around desperately to give some explanation for the cause of CFS. Of the 412 people in the clinical records analyzed from JCM's practice, 71 (17.2%) had laboratory evidence of Epstein–Barr virus infection and 127 (30.8%) stated that their illness began with another virus infection such as influenza or gastroenteritis. Viruses which are known to remain in the body for a long time and become reactivated were therefore an attractive explanation in the 1980s for the increasing number of people with CFS. Epstein–Barr virus (EBV) which causes infectious mononucleosis, cytomegalovirus which causes hepatitis and other infections, human herpes virus types 6 and 7 which affect infants and immunocompromised people, have all been considered interesting candidates as the infection which causes the problem. The difficulty is that most of us have been infected at some time by one or other of these viruses and most of us do not have CFS. Straus (1993) has summarized their role as 'totally innocent bystanders to the illness and its pathophysiological origins'.

A similar story applies to the attempt to link enteroviruses such as Coxsackie virus to the syndrome. This was the virus pursued as a cause in the UK in the 1980s. These viruses are very common and cause outbreaks of infection in children such as hand, foot and mouth disease. They can also cause problems in the CNS with meningitis and cerebellar ataxia, the muscles giving myalgia and the heart, giving rise to myocarditis and pericarditis. With this broad array of diseases, it is not surprising that this common group of viruses was suspected of being the cause of CFS. Studies of antibody titers to Coxsackie B viruses in people with protracted illness with symptoms suggesting CFS showed that about half of them had high titers suggesting the infection as a cause (Calder and Warnock, 1984; Calder et al., 1987). A later study failed to show that this test for the virus was a reliable diagnostic test for CFS in community-based populations (Miller et al., 1991). Reports of the finding of enterovirus RNA sequences in the skeletal muscle and stools of CFS patients (Yousef et al., 1988) have not been confirmed. So the enterovirus link has also proved to be inconsistent.

After the massive breakthrough of discovering that HIV/AIDS was caused by a retrovirus, it was perhaps inevitable that there should be a search in the body fluids of CFS sufferers for the specific retrovirus which 'caused' their illness. In 1991 Defreitas and her colleagues published evidence of HTLV sequences in patients with CFS and it was thought that this discovery might lead to the development of a diagnostic test for CFS. The discovery has not been confirmed by others (Gow et al., 1992). Structures consistent in size, shape and character with a lentivirus were seen under electron microscopy in blood from patients in this clinical series (Holmes et al., 1997), but no other features were confirmed. Other claims of new 'stealth' viruses continue to be made but the problem is that many of these viruses and the antibodies they produce are very prevalent in the community and affect healthy as well as sick people.

However, the role of viruses in the causation of CFS may be more subtle than an attack and destroy policy which leaves behind an imprint detectable by laboratory experiments. Oldstone (1989) has suggested that viruses may reside in cells and yet not produce the classic hallmarks of viral infection. They do not kill the cells and do not elicit an immune response. Rather, they are enabled to establish a long-term presence within cells where they can have a subtle and persistent effect, often by altering a specialized function of the cell, such as the production or secretion of a hormone. It is suggested that diabetes may be caused by such an effect on the insulin-producing cells of the pancreas.

Given the vast number of cells in the body, particularly in the brain, it is altogether possible that such a viral alteration of cell function could play a part in the causation of CFS.

While most people with CFS relate the start of their illness with a viral illness such as influenza or gastroenteritis, this is much more difficult to establish in prospective studies. A prospective study (Wessely et al., 1995) showed no difference in the prevalence of chronic fatigue or CFS six months after exposure to an infectious illness. However, in real populations, if the prevalence of CFS is 0.5% and the mean time to diagnosis is ›5 years, such an association would be extremely difficult to demonstrate apart from epidemic situations.

Immune dysfunction

The interest in a viral causation for the syndrome naturally brought up the issue that it might also be associated with immune dysfunction. Indeed, in the US, the syndrome is called chronic fatigue and immune dysfunction syndrome (CFIDS). The immune system is a complex network of organs (bone marrow, spleen, lymph nodes), cells (lymphocytes, monocytes and macrophages) and molecules (antibodies, complement and cytokines) whose principal function is to protect or defend the body against foreign substances such as viruses, bacteria and pollens. The structure of the immune system is the collection of lymphoid organs in the body connected together by two extensive networks of vessels, the circulatory and lymphatic systems. The communication within the system takes place through the various cells and molecules which circulate in the fluid. Thus, the healthy individual possesses this very complex ability to recognize and destroy any molecule detected by the body which is not recognized as self. This is an extremely complex system but it is made even more complex by the fact that there are interconnections between the immune system and the nervous system mediated by the hypothalamo–pituitary–adrenal axis, cytokines, neuropeptides and neurotransmitters and the autonomic nervous system. This means that all these parts form a continuum which affect each other. Therefore, if you are infected by a virus, the effects may spread to make you tired, depressed or anxious, your hormones are likely to be affected and an imbalance of the autonomic nervous system may give you symptoms, to the extent that it is impossible to tell which came first.

Many studies have looked at the function of the various components of the immune system, comparing the findings with controls, and there have been inconsistent results. Komaroff and Buchwald (1998) reported that the most robust findings have been of increased numbers of CD8+ lymphocytes, depressed numbers of natural killer cells, elevated levels of circulating immune complexes and increased levels of autoantibodies, all evidence of immune activation. On the other hand, Lloyd and his colleagues (1989) reported immune depression with evidence of reduction in T-cell function on skin testing, confirming the original work of Murdoch (1988). Therefore, to summarize, there seem to be no consistent patterns which can be relied upon to confirm the diagnosis of CFS in the individual case although the presence of anergy to an array of antigens such as in the Cell Mediated Immunity Multitest (CMIM) (Institut Merieux 1982) or the presence of a positive autoantibody could be considered as clues where the diagnosis is difficult.

Hypothalamo–pituitary–end organ function

A consistent finding in the study of CFS is that 75% of those affected are female and this has led to questions being asked about whether this might be related to the role of female sex hormones. In the study of 412 people in Dunedin, 68% of the patients were women and 20 of these women stated that their problem had started immediately after a pregnancy. The control of the sex hormones, and those from the thyroid and adrenal glands, is through the pituitary and the hypothalamus and the hypothalamo–pituitary–endocrine gland axis controls the production of hormones. However, the hypothalamus has also important connections upwards to various parts of the midbrain and it is also involved in vital regulatory mechanisms such as the control of temperature, sleep, hunger, thirst and the emotions of fear, rage and motivation. The hypothalamus is also vitally connected to the autonomic nervous system that affects the control of virtually every cell in the body. It is impossible to exaggerate the importance of the hypothalamus and its axes in the maintenance of physical and psychological balance in the adult human being.

The hypothalamic control of the endocrine system is by a series of feedback mechanisms involving the production of hormones in the hypothalamus, pituitary and the thyroid, adrenal, ovarian and testicular glands. In the case of the adrenal gland there are three levels with the hypothalamus producing corticotrophin releasing hormone (CRH), the pituitary gland producing adrenocorticotropic hormone (ACTH), and the adrenal cortex, cortisol. Demitrack and colleagues (1991) demonstrated abnormalities in the hypothalamo–pituitary–adrenal axis in CFS patients with lower urinary excretion of free cortisol and lower evening plasma cortisol levels. ACTH levels were increased, suggesting that the defect in CFS was the production by the hypothalamus of CRH. This was in contrast to work in people with depression where plasma cortisol levels were increased. Other workers (MacHale et al., 1998) have found lower morning and higher evening levels of cortisol in CFS patients as compared to controls and higher ACTH levels in both morning and evening. While these differences were non-significant, the diurnal change in cortisol was significantly less in CFS people and the evening level correlated significantly with measures of general health and physical functioning. They concluded that the results suggested a relationship between adrenocortical function and disability in CFS. Another pointer to a possible mechanism linking fatigue with hypothalamic function came in a study (Barron et al., 1985) of over-trained athletes. This syndrome occurs in athletes exposed to continuous strenuous training. Studies of hypothalamic function showed impaired hormonal responses to insulin-induced hypoglycemia, indicating hypothalamic dysfunction. The same relationship between possible hypothalamic dysfunction and endocrine disturbances has been seen in female ballet dancers and athletes who develop amenorrhea.

The role of impairment in the hypothalamo–pituitary–adrenal axis has not been finally confirmed and has been challenged by contrary results (Young et al., 1998) and the finding of normal salivary cortisol profiles in CFS (Wood et al., 1998). However, there have been trials of low-dose hydrocortisone (Cleare et al., 1999; McKenzie et al., 1998) and fludrocortisone (Peterson et al., 1998) in CFS which have shown some short-term improvement with longer term side effects because the feedback mechanism outlined above makes the therapy difficult to manage. The further evaluation of the role of the hypothalamus in the causation of the symptoms of CFS is yet to be done. However, the mechanisms involved may arise from interference with the neuroendocrine function of the hypothalamus particularly through the control of emotions, sleep and motivation (Bearn and Wessely, 1994). There have also been many interesting observations and speculations concerning the role of neurotransmitters such as 5-Hydroxytryptamine (5HT) which have suggested that symptoms are caused by dysregulation of this compound (Bakheit et al., 1992; Cleare et al., 1995; Sharpe et al., 1997). There have also been neuroimaging studies using advanced techniques such as magnetic resonance imaging (MRI) and single-photon emission tomography (SPET) which have described cerebral white-matter abnormalities in people with CFS and changes in regional cerebral-blood flow (Buchwald et al., 1992).

Given the complicated nature of the relationships between the CNS and the endocrine glands through the 'spaghetti junction' of the hypothalamus, it is unlikely that the symptoms of CFS will ever be understood by studying individuals at this precise chemical and molecular level. However, the research which has been done so far indicates the strong possibility that abnormalities in hypothalamic function or control, possibly initiated by viral infection, may underline the development of the symptoms of CFS. Developing this theme, it has been suggested (Lawrie et al., 1997) that CFS is best understood as a primary disturbance of the sense of effort. They suggest that people with CFS may have to devote more attention to both motor output and somatosensory feedback during exertion, leading to a greater perception of effort and a reduced tolerance of activity. They point to the fact that objective impairment of cognitive function in CFS is impressive evidence of a 'brain-based disturbance of higher function'. This in turn may relate to the viral alteration of cells, referred to above as viral infections, which can cause psychomotor performance impairments even after the resolution of initial symptoms. This may explain the stories of cognitive impairment which most CFS sufferers relate to their physicians but which may not be accompanied by objective evidence.

> Short-term memory can be so poor that they forget the names of good friends. They wake up feeling it is time to retire. Their muscles are extremely weak. Attempts to engage in muscle-strengthening exercises result in days of extreme exhaustion. (Murtagh, 1992)

Is chronic fatigue syndrome a psychological impairment?

Earlier in this chapter we have described the papers of McEvedy and Beard and their contention that the early descriptions of this illness were the result either of mass hysteria or altered medical perception. In most recent outbreaks and in virtually all individual cases, individuals, their families and their doctors raise the question as to whether the cause of their symptoms is 'all in the mind'. The use of this phrase betrays two unfortunate tendencies, the first to split our bodies into physical and mental parts and the second that any cause has to be one or the other and not both. In Chapter 5 we shall examine the societal role of specializations such as psychiatry in controlling the uncertainty of having large numbers of people who have unexplained illness. Here we will confine ourselves to an analysis of the scientific evidence that CFS is a psychological illness.

The term 'functional somatic syndrome' has recently been applied to several related syndromes characterized more by symptoms, suffering and disability than by consistently demonstrable tissue abnormality (Barsky and Borus, 1999; Wessely et al., 1999). These syndromes include multiple chemical sensitivity, the sick-building syndrome, repetition stress injury, the side effects of silicone breast implants, the Gulf War syndrome, chronic whiplash, the irritable bowel syndrome, fibromyalgia and CFS. According to Barsky and Borus, patients with functional somatic syndromes have explicit and highly elaborated self-diagnoses, and their symptoms are often refractory to reassurance, explanation and standard treatment of symptoms. They share similar phenomenologies, high rates of co-occurrence, similar epidemiologic characteristics and higher-than-expected prevalences of psychiatric co-morbidity. Barsky and Borus state that:

although discrete pathophysiologic causes may ultimately be found in some patients with functional somatic syndromes, the suffering of these patients is exacerbated by a self-perpetuating, self-validating cycle in which common, endemic, somatic symptoms are incorrectly attributed to serious abnormality, reinforcing the patient's belief that he or she has a serious disease. Four psychosocial factors propel this cycle of symptom amplification: the belief that one has a serious disease; the expectation that one's condition is likely to worsen; the 'sick role', including the effects of litigation and compensation; and the alarming portrayal of the condition as catastrophic and disabling. The climate surrounding functional somatic syndromes includes sensationalized media coverage, profound suspicion of medical expertise and physicians, the mobilization of parties with a vested self-interest in the status of functional somatic syndromes, litigation and a clinical approach that overemphasizes the biomedical and ignores psychosocial factors. All of these influences exacerbate and perpetuate the somatic distress of patients with functional somatic syndromes, heighten their fears and pessimistic expectations, prolong their disability and reinforce their sick role.

Like McEvedy and Beard (1970a, b), Barsky and Borus (2000) produced a paper review and its arguments seem more political than psychological. Any reference to individual persons affected or different countries would indicate that the approach involves dangerous generalization. For example, in New Zealand there is no litigation and little investigation of any CFS patient and yet the prevalence is similar to that in the US. They deny that they are implying that psychosocial factors initiate the symptoms or are necessarily their primary cause.

> However, once patients are symptomatic, then beliefs, expectations, the sick role and psychological distress become important in amplifying, maintaining and perpetuating these symptoms and in heightening the disability they engender.

One of the major problems about the psychiatric models used in such critiques is that they have no pathophysiological basis and are therefore difficult to prove or refute. This does not necessarily mean that psychiatric models are unable to explain the phenomena. Like most specialties in medicine, the specialty of psychiatry arose from the need to treat and explain the illnesses of special people in a special way, and therefore many of its fundamental principles may seem as quaint as the treatments and explanations in homeopathy, chiropractic or even family medicine to those outside these specialties. However, there is as yet no objective evidence for Freud's superego, ego or id. Nor is there any objective verification of such diagnoses as depression or schizophrenia. The authority of psychiatry has come from the absolute requirement to control people who exhibit abnormal and disturbing behaviors and are, as a result, a danger to themselves, their families and society at large. Like all self-respecting professions, psychiatrists have had to base their assessments and treatments on assumptions or paradigms that few of them question. Like other doctors such as family doctors, their strength lies in the management of individual patients and in the control of their symptoms, with or without the scientific explanations. The decisions made in the course of practicing the specialty, as in family medicine, have been managerial rather than explanatory.

Over the last 50 years, however, the growth in the importance of academic respectability has forced these person-based medical specialties to develop scientific justification around themselves and they have done this by importing science from other disciplines into their techniques and methodologies. Psychiatry has been particularly adept in two areas; psychology and epidemiology. From psychology have come the instruments which now give a measure of so-called objectivity to psychiatric diagnosis. Thus, people can now be labeled authoritatively as psychiatric cases, as depressed, as certain personality types, as not coping, even as fatigued by asking them to fill in self-report questionnaires and having their responses add up to a number which classifies them. This objectification of subjectivity provides a cloak of respectability to a very uncertain area of human behavior and tends to simplify what are very complex behaviors.

Possibly the most florid example of reductionism in the history of medicine has been to reduce human behavior, personality and symptoms to a number through various 'validated' instruments. Once the number has been calculated and abstracted all the individuals who scored 0, 1, 2, 3 and so on are assumed to have more features in common than their differences. Generalizations can then be constructed whereby 'probable psychiatric caseness' is established by scoring at or above a certain level in a 12-question 'instrument' (GHQ-12). Note the allusion to the laboratory in the semantics of this so-called science. Klinkman *et al.* (1998) has shown that misidentification of depression in primary care can be in part an artifact of the use of the psychiatric model of caseness in the primary care setting.

Once a person's story has been converted to a number the science of epidemiology takes over. Epidemiology is the study of the incidence and distribution of diseases and their control and prevention. A great leap has taken place whereby the honest answers of individuals about how they are feeling is converted to a number, then to a disease whose distribution can be measured. This might have been justified in the context of the world where mental illness is treated but can it be extended to make sense of the whole world? The attempt has been made and this has led to a classification of psychiatric diagnosis, the *Diagnostic and Statistical Manual of Mental Disorders* (American Psychiatric Association, 1994) which includes agreed criteria for many symptom presentations, some of which overlap with the criteria for CFS.

Thus, when modern psychiatrists are asked to assess people with the symptoms of CFS, they seem to be able to make authoritative diagnoses from this classification. However, we have to remember that this diagnosis is based on the subjective response of the person affected. Traditionally, psychoanalysis has used these responses to help the individual affected. Medawar (1984) argued that 'a psychoanalytical interpretation weaves around the patient a well-tailored personal myth within the plot of which the subject's thoughts and behaviour seem only natural.' This very personal interaction between consenting adults has now been depersonalized and standardized through the processes described above and we are now asked to accept the evidence as scientific.

One of the major problems faced by those attempting to explain the symptoms of CFS as a psychiatric illness is the deep resentment which this position arouses in patient groups. The reason often given for this resentment is hostility to psychological, as opposed to physical, explanations for illness, but it may be that the resentment is itself evidence of the lack of rigor of the evidence. It may be that what a person writes on a questionnaire or a symptom inventory can only be interpreted with the consent of the individual patient and not by assigning a numerical value. Perhaps the instruments refined in 'psychiatric' populations cannot be reliably used in 'fatigued' populations.

So we are left with a conflict in the research about the possible causes of CFS because those who accept the psychiatric basis of classification appear to believe that there then is no further need to search for an organic cause for the problem, and to upgrade the diagnosis. In doing this they seem to believe that a psychiatric diagnosis is an organic cause or at least its equivalent. It also seems to suggest that such a psychiatric classification is final which it was never meant to be. The statement that someone has a depressive illness is merely a psychiatric refinement of what they feel and has no causal implications. The same could be said for the statements that people have somatization disorder, or neurasthenia or hysteria. These are also merely statements about how a psychiatrist explains to the patient and his family why it is that she/he has these particular symptoms. These psychometric classifications give very disappointing results in the prediction and treatment of psychiatric morbidities such as depression. It would suggest that an oversimplification of a complex process is at work (Rost et al., 2000).

However, it is a paradox that the psychiatrists who seem to deprecate the search for an organic cause for CFS by suggesting that belief in an organic cause is associated with a poor prognosis (Joyce et al., 1997) seem to lead the search for an organic cause such as a hypothalamic one. This suggests that they too believe that a psychosocial model alone is too limited for an understanding of CFS.

Like Epstein et al. (1999) we believe this should be a biopsychosocial model with contributions from the patient-centered clinical method in which all significant illnesses are seen as multilevel disorders involving bodily function, emotions and social relationships. If the psychological factors playing a part in that complex process in CFS are to be evaluated in research, they have to be seen as only a part of the whole. There is good evidence for suggesting this because, while psychogenic factors are undoubtedly important in CFS, most studies show that co-morbid psychological illnesses occur in only around 50%, suggesting that they are the result of coping with the difficulties of the symptoms rather than its cause.

However, an important condition of the adoption of this model is that it will only be successful in healing if the explanations have the full consent of the person affected. Because psychiatry originally developed in the days of the physical restraint and compulsory care of psychosis, it does not come from a patient-centered tradition, and has a past which most of society is still coming to terms with. The current reality of living with CFS is that the suggestion of seeing a psychiatrist is a statement which means that no disease exists which, in turn, means that the person will have no access to resources for recovery and that judgment, guilt, blame and shame have to be borne directly by the person with the symptoms.

The value of psychiatry as a co-operating discipline in the management of CFS is to help people or their relatives with their emotional and psychological suffering which in turn may persuade them to accept symptomatic treatments. However, if it is to be helpful, psychiatry as a specialization, like family medicine, has to abandon the high ground of absolute certainty in diagnosis in order to earn the right to participate in the delivery of an explanation for the disorder. This involves a reorientation of psychiatric practice toward care of the patient rather than the illusion of accurate classification of disease. Until that happens there will be no meaningful progress in psychiatric research into CFS.

From disappointment to clarification: future development of research into chronic fatigue syndrome

There is no doubt that the conclusions drawn by some on the research into CFS so far is that no great light has been shed on the problem which will assist the doctor who sits and listens to the typical story of disabling symptoms which have destroyed a life, a family and a career. However, the search for one 'cause' has to be put in perspective because the discovery of such a cause will have its application at one level of the multilevel disorder. For example, if a 'stealth' virus had been consistently found in all CFS sufferers, what improvement would this have effected in the management of the individual? It could be argued that the main improvements would have been in the attitude of doctors and in the morale of patients, but it seems odd that human kindness should be conditional on biological differences.

Unfortunately, having a Down's syndrome child was not made significantly easier by the discovery of a trisomy in chromosome 21 (Lejeune et al., 1959). Although this study will be credited with discovering the cause of Down's syndrome, this certainly did not eliminate the effects of having the syndrome. It could be argued that normalization of intellectually handicapped people generally, the treatment of serous otitis media as the major cause of deafness or the early identification of thyroid deficiency have contributed much more to improving the quality of life of the Down's syndrome person than knowing that they have an extra chromosome, the 'cause' of the diagnosis.

Research into CFS as a medical entity during the 20th century, has largely been a battle for the supremacy of models in which the role of persons with CFS has been the supply of bodily fluids and questionnaires. The proponents of the biomedical model have produced a significant body of historical description and current research which at least challenges the statement that there is no scientific proof that CFS exists as a separate disease entity. However, the disappointment with the results of the research simply reflects the fact that no single biological difference exists in people with CFS which separates them from the rest of humanity. Because of the anachronistic and positivist rules governing the funding and publication of these scientific battles, CFS seems destined to be classified, almost by default, as a minor psychiatric disorder of no great import. However, the combatants do not seem to realize that in the real world the prevailing opinion is that the public regards the problem as common, important and often serious and is demanding research to provide a solution. The problem is that current research methods seem incapable of providing answers.

So which directions do we take in research?

The first requirement is to center it on the subject of the inquiry, the person with the problem, and in the wider community where they develop the problem. Observing these people over a long number of years reinforces the opinion that most of those who present in this way are normal, healthy people who suddenly become ill and then commence a long trek back to some form of health. Given the prevalence of 500 per 100 000 or 0.5%, it is difficult though not impossible to obtain the information that sets the problem in its context. This is made much more difficult by the disdain in which individual case reporting is held. The recognition and study of symptoms and their management will always be the foundation of any valid research into CFS.

The second point is that proof of causality is not a necessary outcome of any research into CFS. McWhinney (1991) has said that we must move away from a simple view of causality in our research efforts.

What we think of as causal agents may simply be acting as triggers that release some process already inherent in the organism. Whether the process is activated by the trigger depends on the state of the organism at the time. The final state of the organism, moreover, will depend less on the causal agent than on its own complex responses.

This point is illustrated by a study of patients with headache (Headache Study Group of the University of Western Ontario, 1986) presenting to general practitioners in which the strongest predictor of resolution at 12 months was the patient's statement after the first visit that there had been a good opportunity

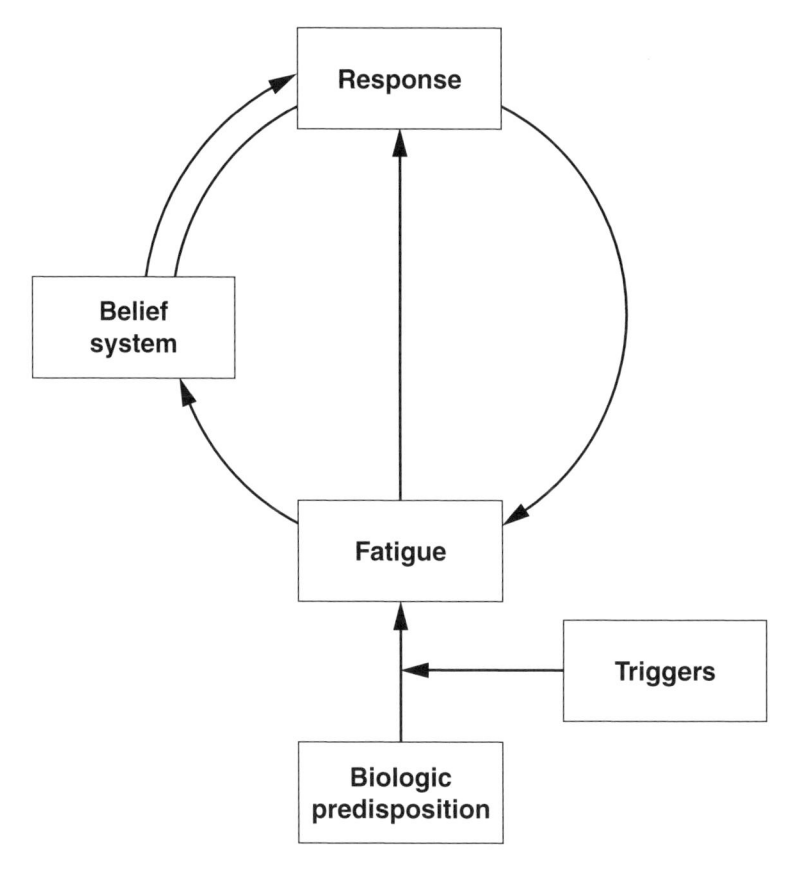

Figure 3.1 An explanatory model for the mechanism of chronic fatigue (adapted and used with the permission of Sage Publications Inc.).

to discuss the problem with the doctor. This is used to produce an explanatory model of headache which can be modified to apply to the CFS patient (*see* Figure 3.1). The triggers indicated by the 412 people in the Dunedin clinical series (Murdoch, 2000) varied from EBV (71), other virus (127), pregnancy (20), stress (23), chemicals (14), bacterial infection (16), operation/anesthetic (16), to none (124). It is altogether possible that any trigger could catapult a human being into the state of CFS. What ought to be the subject of our research is the nature of the defining characteristics of a person who is subject to this transformation. This will involve the production of descriptive and qualitative research which have their own standards of rigor.

Conclusion: still a piece of nonsense, Dr Rose?

This chapter has been necessarily long because there has been much research done especially over the past 15 years. While this has reached no definite conclusion, we are sure that even Dr Rose could not regard it as a piece of nonsense. Indeed, Wendy and her family might have felt a great deal better if he had been able to give them a short summary of the research done so far. There seems to be enough in the scientific literature to persuade even the most serious doubter of the possibility that CFS may yet be recognized as a disease in its own right. What is required is the will to recognize the illness as different and to come up with a unifying scientific hypothesis which will further define the problem and the characteristics which cause it to persist in some and clear up in others.

References

Acheson ED (1959) The clinical syndrome variously called benign myalgic encephalomyelitis, Iceland disease and epidemic neuromyasthenia. *Am J Med.* **26**: 569–95.

American Psychiatric Association (1994) *Diagnostic and Statistical Manual of Mental Disorders* (4e). American Psychiatric Association, Washington DC.

Bakheit AM, Behan PO, Dinan TG, Gray CE and O'Keane V (1992) Possible upregulation of hypothalamic 5HT receptors in patients with post-viral fatigue syndrome. *BMJ.* **304**: 1010–12.

Barron JL, Noakes TD, Levy W, Smith C and Millar RP (1985) Hypothalamic dysfunction in overtrained athletes. *J Clin Endocrinol Metab.* **60**: 803–6.

Barsky AJ and Borus JF (1999) Functional somatic syndromes: a review. *Ann Intern Med.* **130**: 910–21.

Barsky AJ and Borus JF (2000) Functional somatic syndromes: in response. *Ann Intern Med.* **132**: 327.

Bearn J and Wessely S (1994) Neurobiological aspects of the chronic fatigue syndrome. *Eu J Clin Invest.* **24**: 79–90.

Buchwald D, Cheney PR, Peterson DL *et al.* (1992) A chronic illness characterized by fatigue, neurologic and immunologic disorders, and active human herpes virus type 6 infection. *Ann Intern Med.* **116**: 103–13.

Cleare AJ, Heap E, Malhi GS *et al.* (1999) Low-dose hydrocortisone in chronic fatigue syndrome: a randomised cross-over trial. *Lancet,* **353**: 455–8.

Cleare AJ, Bearn J, Allain T *et al.* (1995) Contrasting neuroendocrine responses in depression and chronic fatigue syndrome. *J Affect Disord.* **35**: 283–9.

Calder BD and Warnock PJ (1984) Coxsackie B infection in a Scottish general practice. *J R Coll Gen Pract.* **34**: 15–19.

Calder BD, Warnock PJ, McCartney RA and Bell EJ (1987) Coxsackie B viruses and the post-viral syndrome: a prospective study in general practice. *J R Coll Gen Pract.* **37**: 11–14.

Defreitas E, Hilliard B, Cheney PR *et al.* (1991) Retroviral sequences related to human T-lymphotropic virus type II in patients with chronic immune dysfunction syndrome. *Proc Nat Acad Sci.* **88**: 2922–6.

Demitrack M, Dale J, Straus SE *et al.* (1991) Evidence for impaired activation of the hypothalamic–pituitary–adrenal axis in patients with chronic fatigue syndrome. *J Clin Endocrin Metab.* **73**: 1224–34.

Editorial: Epidemic Malaise. (1970) *BMJ.* **1**: 1–2.

Engel GL (1988) How much longer must medicine's science be bound by a seventeenth century world view? In: KL White (ed.) *The Task of Medicine: dialogue at Wickenburg.* The Henry Kaiser Family Foundation, Menlo Park, CA.

Epstein RM, Quill TE and McWhinney IR (1999) Somatization reconsidered. Incorporating the patient's experience of illness. *Arch Fam Med.* **159**: 215–22.

Feinstein AR (1970) What kind of basic science for clinical medicine? *NEJM.* **283**: 847–52.

Gow JW, Simpson K, Schliephake A *et al.* (1992) Search for retrovirus in the chronic fatigue syndrome. *J Clin Pathol.* **45**: 1058–61.

Headache Study Group of the University of Western Ontario (1986) Predictors of outcome in headache patients presenting to family physicians: a one year prospective study. *Headache.* **26**: 285–94.

Holmes MJ, Diack DS, Easingwood RA, Cross JP and Carlisle B (1997) Electron microscopic immunocytological profiles in chronic fatigue syndrome. *J Psychiatr Res.* **31**: 115–22.

Howie JGR (1991) Refining questions and hypotheses. In: PG Norton, M Stewart, F Tudiver *et al.* (eds) *Primary Care Research: traditional and innovative approaches.* Sage Publications, Newbury Park, CA.

Institut Merieux (1982) *Multitest CMI: a skin test for evaluation of cell-mediated immunity.* Edico Publicis, Lyon, France.

Joyce J, Hotopf M and Wessely S (1997) The prognosis of chronic fatigue and chronic fatigue syndrome: a systematic review. *Q J Med.* **90**: 223–33.

Klinkman MS, Coyne JC, Gallo S and Schwenk TL (1998) False positives, false negatives, and the validity of the diagnosis of major depression in primary care. *Arch Fam Med.* **7**: 451–61.

Komaroff AL and Buchwald DS (1998) Chronic fatigue syndrome: an update. *Ann Rev Med.* **49**: 1–13.

Kuhn TS (1967) *The Structure of Scientific Revolutions.* University of Chicago Press, Chicago, IL.

Lawrie SM, Machale SM, Power MJ and Goodwin GM (1997) Is the chronic fatigue syndrome best understood as a primary disturbance of the sense of effort? *Psychol Med.* **27**: 995–9.

Lejeune J, Gautier M and Turpin R (1959) Etudes des chromosomes somatiques de neuf enfants mongoliens. *Comptes Rendus Hebdomadaires des Seances de L'academie des Sciences.* **248**: 1721–2.

Lipkowski ZJ (1988) Somatization: the concept and its clinical application. *Am J Psychiatry.* **145**: 1358–68.

Lloyd AR, Wakefield D, Boughton CR and Dwyer JM (1989) Immunological abnormalities in the chronic fatigue syndrome. *Med J Aust.* **151**: 122–4.

MacHale SM, Cavanagh JT, Bennie J et al. (1998) Diurnal variation of adrenocortical activity in chronic fatigue syndrome. *Neuropsychobiology.* **38**: 213–17.

Mackenzie J (1919) *The Future of Medicine.* Hodder & Stoughton, London, UK.

May PGR, Donnan SPB, Ashton JR, Ogilvie MM and Rolles CJ (1980) Personality and medical perception in benign myalgic encephalomyelitis. *Lancet.* **2**: 1122–4.

McEvedy CP and Beard AW (1970a) Concept of benign myalgic encephalomyelitis. *BMJ.* **1**: 11–15.

McEvedy CP and Beard AW (1970b) Royal Free epidemic of 1955: a reconsideration. *BMJ.* **1**: 7–11.

McKenzie R, O'Fallon A, Dale J et al. (1998) Low-dose hydrocortisone for treatment of chronic fatigue syndrome: a randomized controlled trial. *JAMA.* **280**: 1061–6.

McWhinney IR (1984) Changing models: the impact of Kuhn's theory on medicine. *Fam Pract.* **1**(1): 3–8.

McWhinney IR (1991) Primary care research in the next twenty years. In: PG Norton, M Stewart, F Tudiver et al. (eds) *Primary Care Research: traditional and innovative approaches.* Sage Publications, Newbury Park, CA.

Medewar P (1984) *Science and Literature in Pluto's Republic.* Oxford University Press, Oxford, UK.

Medical Staff of the Royal Free Hospital (1957) An outbreak of encephalomyelitis in the Royal Free Hospital Group, London, in 1955. *BMJ.* **2**: 895–904.

Miller NA, Carmichael HA, Calder BD et al. (1991) Antibody to Coxsackie B virus in diagnosing post-viral fatigue syndrome. *BMJ.* **302**: 140–3.

Murdoch JC (1988) Cell-mediated immunity in patients with myalgic encephalomyelitis syndrome. *N Z Med J.* **101**: 511–12.

Murdoch JC (1997) Mackenzie's puzzle: the cornerstone of teaching and research in general practice. *Br J Gen Pract*. **47**: 656–8.

Murtagh J (1992) *Cautionary Tales: authentic case histories from medical practice*. McGraw-Hill Book Company, Sydney, Australia.

Odegaard CE (1986) *Dear Doctor: a personal letter to a physician*. The Henry Kaiser Family Foundation, Menlo Park, CA.

Oldstone MBA (1989) Viral alteration of cell function. *Sci Am*. **August**: 34–40.

Peterson PK, Pheley A, Schroeppel J *et al.* (1998) A preliminary placebo-controlled cross-over trial of fludrocortisone for chronic fatigue syndrome. *Arch Intern Med*. **158**: 908–14.

Ramsay AM (1978) General discussion. Epidemic neuromyasthenia 1934–77: current approaches. *Postgrad Med J*. **54**: 743.

Richmond C (1989) Myalgic encephalomyelitis, Princess Aurora, and the wandering womb. *BMJ*. **298**: 1295–6.

Rost K, Nutting P, Smith J *et al.* (2000) The role of competing demands in the treatment provided primary care patients with major depression. *Arch Fam Med*. **9**: 150–4.

Sharpe M, Hawton K, Clements K and Cowen PJ (1997) Increased brain serotonin function in men with chronic fatigue syndrome. *BMJ*. **315**: 164–5.

Shorter E (1992) Somatization at the end of the twentieth century. In: E Shorter *From Paralysis to Fatigue*. The Free Press, New York.

Straus SE (1993) Studies of herpes virus infection in chronic fatigue syndrome. *Ciba Found Symp*. **173**: 132–9.

Wessely S, Chalder T, Hirsch S *et al.* (1995) Post-infectious fatigue: prospective cohort study in primary care. *Lancet*. **345**: 1333–8.

Wessely S, Nimnuan C and Sharpe M (1999) Functional somatic syndromes: one or many? *Lancet*. **354**: 936–9.

Wood B, Wessely S, Papadopoulos A, Poon L and Checkley S (1998) Salivary cortisol profiles in chronic fatigue syndrome. *Neuropsychobiology*. **37**: 1–4.

Young AH, Sharpe M, Clements A *et al.* (1998) Basal activity of the hypothalamic–pituitary–adrenal axis in patients with the chronic fatigue syndrome. *Biol Psychiatry*. **43**: 236–7.

Yousef GE, Bell EJ, Mann GF *et al.* (1988) Chronic enterovirus infection in patients with post-viral fatigue syndrome. *Lancet*. **1**: 146–50.

Understanding the whole person

Case study

Wendy Jones was married at 22 to Willie. The marriage appeared satisfactory. Both were patients in Dr Rose's practice but Willie was seen by Dr Rose only occasionally, primarily for minor work-related injuries. Wendy had done well at school but having met Willie in her last year, she had opted not to go to university. Instead, she got work in a medical laboratory and had become a competent and highly skilled laboratory technician. She worked in a research unit along with about ten other staff. She had been aware that the job was not going to develop any further because her technical training was insufficient to allow her to lead research. Other technicians who had been in the unit for many years were not doing anything more than she was. She was bored and wondered where her life was going from there.

Wendy had discussed having children with Dr Rose at the appointments for the contraceptive pill. She and Willie had been delaying having their first child in order to concentrate on reducing the mortgage on their house, but given the dissatisfaction at work, they decided to have the first child, and she had gone back to work eight weeks later. Her mother helped out with the childcare and it was only well into her second pregnancy that she had given up paid work. Just two months before the birth, Willie had lost his job and this was stressful to them both as they had planned on living on one income until both children were at school.

Her father had been most upset when Willie had gone to him asking for money to start his own business and let him know in no uncertain terms that he had always felt that his daughter was too good for Willie and that she would have been better never marrying him. Willie, in turn, declared Wendy's father a real snob and made it clear that they were going to be independent from any help, even his mother-in-law's care of the children. Willie's father was no help at all as he was unemployed and had separated from Willie's mother when Willie was 12 years old, having fallen for a younger woman. He could not understand why Willie wanted to start his own business as he could go on the government unemployment assistance 'until something turned up'. He had been waiting for something to turn up for years and was known to drink too much. Willie's mother was, in Wendy's words, 'a bitter woman', who had refused her estranged husband a divorce but nevertheless worked hard to support Willie, her only son.

Wendy tried to maintain a semblance of normality with all concerned throughout the pregnancy and birth but had to do a fair amount of manipulating to keep the warring parties apart. Sleep became an increasing problem towards the end and while she was breastfeeding. Worries about money seemed to dominate the conversation between the couple since the job loss. Though Willie tried to keep a brave face on things, she knew that the bank manager was having increasing problems about the size of their bank overdraft.

However, in spite of all the financial problems and familial discord, Wendy gained immense satisfaction from motherhood and her time at home with the children. That is, she did until the flu that preceded the cascade of symptoms that she now has.

In the last chapter we were able to observe the struggle which has ensued to prove whether CFS is a real disease or not. This desire by both patients and doctors to have the illness qualify for inclusion in 'the list of illnesses to be taken seriously' demonstrates just how doctor- and diagnosis-centered our modern health services are. However, in the time that it takes to reach a verdict on whether a legitimate disease is present, the life of the person moves on, and unfortunately, the reluctance to treat the problem seriously may contribute to the severity of the condition and to the effect which it has on the individual and the family. In the practice of patient-centered medicine the understanding of the person who has the symptoms becomes the key to applying treatment whether or not there is agreement on a diagnosis. We have argued in Chapter 1 that there is ample evidence of adequate criteria on which to make a diagnosis. In Chapter 2 we have heard clearly the witness of a legitimate illness experience. Chapter 3 has given evidence of a number of explanatory mechanisms for that illness. The absolute proof of these mechanisms must await the outcome of further research. However, we believe that the crucial issue in the healing of the patient lies not so much in the correct understanding of the science as in the understanding of the person who has CFS. For the remainder of this book we will therefore concentrate on the person and their connections with family and society, and the task for this chapter is to understand the varying effects of the stage of the illness, the role of the coping mechanisms of the person and their family, and the contribution of the person's place in the lifecycle.

In looking at these further issues, there will inevitably be overlap between the theoretical models described by Stewart and her colleagues (Stewart *et al.*,

1995). It seems to us impossible to separate out the illness experience from the whole person or from the aspect of finding common ground. We believe that it is useful to base this understanding under three headings: the stage of the illness, family ways of coping, and the stage of the lifecycle. Some might argue that the first, the stage of the illness, should be discussed as part of the illness experience. It is placed here because the length of the illness in CFS is such that it almost creates a new version of the lifecycle and so we felt that a discussion of these aspects fitted here rather than in Chapter 2.

The circumstances of each case of CFS will differ with respect to the individual who is affected and the context of her or his circumstances at the time of illness. This is regardless of what might ensue from the research into CFS with respect to agreement on what constitutes a case, its prevalence and the proof of causation. The majority of reports indicate that the illness is most prevalent in women in their 40s, in Latinos in Chicago, US and in lower socioeconomic groups. In addition, although CFS can strike at virtually any time, the evidence is that CFS is an illness that continues for some time (Jason *et al.*, 1999). In the Chicago study, those with the illness had a much higher rate of unemployment and being on sickness benefit compared to a control group with no illness. The study of 70 people with CFS done in Dunedin (Murdoch and Bradshaw 1984) described the interference in family and working life as those affected struggled with the symptoms and the lack of support given to them by family and colleagues. Thus, by the time people with CFS are studied, they may well have gone through many stages of illness. It is impossible to tell how much of their health status is the result of CFS or of the difficulties into which CFS has led them through the stress of symptoms or unemployment or family difficulties. Chronic illness and unremitting symptoms will, of themselves, produce stress, reactive depression and unhappiness and one role of the family doctor is to bear witness to the happier days when the person was healthy. For some reason Dr Rose seems incapable of doing this, perhaps because he does not consider it part of his role as a physician.

The criteria for CFS described in Chapter 1 have been very valuable to help delineate the common features of the illness, its prevalence and outcome and research into possible causes. It is important, however, to recognize that the course of the illness in individuals will be unique. McWhinney (1989) has urged an 'acquaintance with particulars' whereby the family physician, while being guided by the generalities of illness such as CFS, also pays attention to the context in which the illness has developed. The illness that Wendy has developed has been difficult for all the reasons that have been described. However, what compounds an already difficult illness is the fact that it has developed against a background of family conflict, professional development and disappointment, pregnancy and childbirth. It is impossible to separate which of these might have been important determinants of the outcome for this person at this stage of her life.

Such variations on the theme are as numerous as there are persons with CFS and the end result will be equally varied. At each stage of our lives, all of us are undergoing change in physical, psychological or emotional terms, or are needed as carers or supporters of families or are studying and starting careers. There is no 'identikit picture' of the typical CFS sufferer which will automatically help us to understand the individual sufferer, but there are themes which underline its development at various stages.

In this chapter we will describe the problems encountered using descriptions from the literature and from unpublished material from work with New Zealand patients. Much of what will be described will be anecdotal and we make no apology for that. A vital role of the professional carer of the CFS patient is to listen to the individual story in much the same way as Dr Rose should have listened to Wendy. We hope that this will result in the physician understanding the whole person who is not just an isolated person, but a person in community and mostly as part of a family unit, a unit that needs as much understanding and support as the patient.

The variations on the theme of CFS that will be encountered from patient to patient are dictated by three variants. These are the stage of the illness, the way in which the individual and the family has coped with the illness and the stages of the lifecycle during which the illness became a problem.

The stage of the illness

Because CFS as a diagnosis has only recently become recognized, a special problem which people with the illness have is that they may have to spend a long time without recognition. During this time they were people with somatization or unexplained somatic symptoms. This is a long time, indeed long enough for some to forget what it was like to be well. These people describe various stages of the illness.

Stage one: the crash

Like in a road accident, people with CFS use the term 'crash' to describe their experience. Most have the experience of an acute illness which leaves them weak and reeling like most of us who are in the throes of a viral illness. Family doctors and relatives never cease to be amazed at the way normal, intelligent and reasonable adults can exhibit helpless, confused and infantile behaviors within a few hours of developing a simple viral illness such as influenza. The only consolation is the assurance that can be given that this is a five-day wonder and that all can look forward to the next week when the awful symptoms will have disappeared. The difference with the CFS patient is that, by definition, the symptoms have to last for six months before the problem can be diagnosed with any authority, and then only if the person is fortunate enough to meet a physician who is able to give the diagnosis. The process of the crash usually does as much if not more harm than the virus or other factor that has caused it. In this stage, the person with the illness goes through a period of time when they seem totally out of control, and where they feel physically and emotionally wrecked. The actual problem is poorly understood by those who have not experienced it and they assume the onset to be gradual as in most cases of simple fatigue.

> Two days before Easter of 1984 I was in bed with a bad flu; high temp, etc. The doctor prescribed penicillin but from that day on my normally fit, healthy body slowly started to seize up.

This description underlines one of the differences between doctors and patients in their understanding of CFS. People with CFS almost always remember the point at which their life changed, and they are often irritated by the fact that their doctors do not seem to remember what they were like before the illness struck. It is almost as though some doctors modify the past in the light of the current so-called 'psyche problems' and deny their previous sense of normality. One of the problems, of course, is that many of those affected are in an age group that has had little experience either of illness or of the medical system and a significant number complain that they, as persons, have received little attention. This attention to individual particulars about the patient ought to be one of the functions of the personal doctor. Stephens (1982) quotes Meyer as saying that there are conditions which the physician cannot diagnose without knowing the patient's name and there is certainly a need to know and understand the biography of the person who is lying wounded in this crash. Although most of the time we talk of such particulars in the context of those who have been well becoming sick, it is also important to remember that those who have been sick or who have somatized in the past also require this attention to particulars. There is no evidence that psychiatric or somatization disorder confers immunity to CFS or any other illness.

However, most people who have recently become ill enjoy a honeymoon period and receive a lot of interest from their health professionals at this point and there is much questioning, much examining and much bloodletting, usually all with negative results. Then the hand-washing (its not my fault you are still ill) and the hand waving (why don't you go see someone else) starts. Modern doctors are very intolerant of negative results but tend to get excited if they think something 'serious' or unusual is there to be diagnosed. Common early problems in CFS are a fast pulse rate and palpitations, profound weakness simulating stroke or early multiple sclerosis (MS), abdominal pain and diarrhea. Some are admitted acutely to hospital to coronary care units and surgical and gynecological wards. One patient, a nurse who had become a farmer, wrote:

> My initial symptoms developed some weeks after falling over with a container of herbicide on my back. I thought that the symptoms of sternum tenderness and muscle pain were due to injuries sustained in the fall. Eventually, digging in the garden became too difficult and energy levels decreased. I experienced odd bouts of diarrhea accompanied by explosive bowel wind for no apparent reason. Some months later I developed a tennis elbow which was a nuisance but did not cause much of a problem because it was treated successfully by my GP. The following week I developed tachycardia and palpitations, shortness of breath, stiff neck and painful left shoulder. These symptoms did not worry me but then I experienced weak hands and arms and that did worry me! After resting for ten days, and I mean bedrest, there was no improvement and I consulted my GP. He was concerned enough to have me admitted to hospital for several days to check on the heart situation and probably to rest, but at this point a definitive diagnosis was not made. After hospitalization which included being connected to a heart monitor, I was prescribed a beta blocker.

She then describes in detail the development of the criteria decided a year or two later by the CDCs and also comments on the problems raised by her accurate observations.

> As the weeks went by I continued to get new symptoms and shed others. My GP told me that I was doing well but I felt otherwise and asked for a referral through to you (JCM) as I was sure I had ME. This was not based on intuition but on knowledge gained over the weeks of my illness. I had read a number of good studies which contained much that my medical books didn't; the nearest I could get there was multiple sclerosis. I kept a diary for a while to keep an account of the changing symptom pattern, an exercise that was frowned upon by my doctor and my medical friends. They apparently thought that this would increase my anxiety state.

So it seems that Dr Alan Rose's approach to Wendy's problem is not all that uncommon and the experience of many patients is that doctors seem to demand a cause in exchange for their continuing interest. This leads us into the more dangerous second phase for the longer the doctor keeps telling the patient that there is nothing wrong, the more the person's life falls apart.

Stage two: chronic illness without a label

The doctors' hands are perceived to be washed clean as the bloods are all normal and the specialists' reports are all reassuring to the doctors. The farmer nurse's physician writes:

> This lady became unwell suddenly in April 1985 and presented with palpitations. She also had developed panic attacks at that stage. I admitted her to hospital for observation. On continuous monitoring no changes were seen. Unfortunately another patient in the unit had a cardiac arrest and this caused a lot of concern and anxiety to the patient. I sent her to see Dr X who checked her neurological state and found that she had a fear of multiple sclerosis. He concluded that the tachycardia, the fear, the anxiety, the panic attacks and hyperventilation establishes fairly clearly that this is a 'functional' complaint. He felt that it would be a disservice to her to do lumbar punctures etc. to exclude MS at this stage.

At some point here the four-lane highway which is the path to a diagnosis in modern primary medical care comes to a sudden halt and we enter a difficult phase. Faced with the difficulty of saying that he does not know, a neurologist gives the patient a nonsensical 'fear of MS' diagnosis and decides not to do the investigations that would either confirm or allay her fear. This is almost as insulting as the words of a doctor to a 28-year-old art curator.

> I would go back every three months or so complaining of being tired or having the flu ... I was surprised when this doctor I had been going to for three years suggested that all I needed was a man. I felt that, after running the usual glandular fever tests and blood counts several times which revealed no apparent signs of illness, she gave up on me.

This stage is marked by the emotional and psychological consequences of a long-term unnamed chronic illness and people learn not to be too honest about the way they feel. Sandy, our farmer nurse, remarks:

> Routine tests appeared normal so the illness was seen to be functional and so particularly with women, there tends to be a bias towards a neurosis-type diagnosis. Once thus diagnosed and if the CFS is severe, particularly the psychological symptoms, there is unlikely to be another avenue explored as to the cause of the illness. I personally wasn't quite in this situation but only because I didn't tell my GP every symptom I experienced, particularly the depth of the depression experienced. This was bad enough to warrant medication but I found other ways of coping with it.

There is no doubt that in this stage of the illness the person with CFS is forced to cope with very difficult symptoms and circumstances, and there is a need for doctors to understand their methods of coping and the doctors' own coping strategies.

The difficulty revealed in the latter by the comments of CFS patients is that doctors' help-providing abilities seem to be limited to a medical model which is usually based on the assumption that affected individuals put themselves into the care of doctors who are then responsible for both the problem and the solution. There is nothing more comforting to a patient than to hear the doctors say that they know what is wrong and will put things right. However, the experience in CFS is that this offer does not come because there is a refusal to give the diagnosis and, as a consequence, the sick role. Individuals are only given this relief from the burden of their illness as long as it is 'physical'. When the illness is functional or psychological the person is perceived as being not only responsible for the problem and the solution, but is also judged and found lacking in their personhood. We find ourselves in this situation because most doctors believe that they ought to be able to give a 'scientifically' valid diagnosis and treatment for every patient who sees them. However, if the doctor cannot accept the diagnosis of CFS and knows of no treatment for it, the people affected do not qualify for the medical model. This seems to perplex many doctors. Sandy's physician, a decent man by any standards, expressed the problem in his referral letter.

> I would be interested in hearing your findings for I still have difficulty in deciding on these patients with ME as I am not aware of any conclusive test to help distinguish these cases.

These difficulties experienced by generalists have traditionally been solved by referring the patient to a specialist but the problem is that there are no specialists in CFS. In the absence of tests there are various diagnostic categories into which such misfits are placed but seldom is this a category that is agreed between doctor and patient. The result is that there is discomfort at every meeting and the term 'heartsink' has been used to describe those who persist in having symptoms without a diagnosis from the doctor. Doctors are genuinely upset by such patients but it is interesting that most of the studies on heartsink are aimed at the patient, not the doctor whose heart is sinking.

So why does the absence of a diagnosis have such a disastrous effect on the patient–doctor consultation? Cassell (1991) has indicated that a major problem is the conflict between the kind of knowledge by which physicians know disease and the kind of knowledge by which they know and act on their patients as particular individuals. Given the choice between being diagnostically correct and believing the patient, most doctors will choose the former and neglect the latter. But note how concern for being diagnostically correct is very selective. The doctor described above had difficulty because he lacked certainty in deciding the diagnostic criteria for CFS but he was quite willing to believe the fatuous 'fear of MS' from a neurologist.

There should be a maximum of six months lead-time from the development of such distressing symptoms to the point of diagnosis. Perhaps the length of time without a diagnosis could be avoided if doctors could understand that patients are also intolerant of uncertainty and if there was a discussion on the likely diagnosis in every consultation. The encouragement of a written agenda prepared by patients for the consultations might help to provide a basis for such communication (McKinley and Middleton, 1999).

Stage three: chronic illness with the label of chronic fatigue syndrome

When the person who fulfils the criteria of CFS is given the label, the relief is palpable. Concentration on the burden of proof can now give way to concentration on lifting the burden of illness and the process can move on to the stage of management as will be discussed in Chapter 7. It is a bit like resolving a political crisis. Both parties, doctor and patient, agree to work together on the management of life goals as well as daily tasks. Disputes on diagnosis are such a waste of time in the long term. We can move on to a reassessment of current lifestyle and the management of active illness. People with CFS are unlikely to still be in high-pressure jobs by the time they are diagnosed but there is the issue of managing together their aspirations, personal and societal hopes, fears and expectations given that they can no longer be productive. A major issue is the rebuilding of self-confidence. CFS wreaks havoc with the self-esteem. Nor are they likely to have the high social status that they may be used to, and help has to be given with access to the rehabilitative benefits available from the social services.

Stage four: recovery with relapse

As has been said above, the experience in New Zealand regarding recovery seems to be much more positive than in other parts of the world. However, with recovery come additional problems as often those who have been through this experience are lacking in confidence with respect to their physical abilities. Relapses will often occur unexpectedly. For example, students who have relapses under stress find examinations a major problem. One student had occasions of total loss of recall and reported the inability to recall anything. This was not associated with anxiety or concern. She just stopped thinking and that included worrying. But she also reported one examination when the memory came back about 40 minutes into the exam.

> Like someone had given me a memory injection, it all came back and I passed with an A.

The doctor who is interested in providing a service to such patients will be asked about issues of relapse prevention and relapse management. For example:

- can a triathlete get back into competition?
- how can a recovered child/young adult manage the societal and self-induced demands of career development and socialization?
- will they need to be 'careful about their health' for the rest of their lives?
- is it 'unreasonable for a young person to want to work full-time, play social sport, socialize one or two nights a week and study seven hours a week' without compromising their health?

The most important issue here is dealing honestly and professionally with the person and making sure that they still understand the principles of self-management (*see* Chapter 7).

> Kate (22) had the experience of crashing after 10 years of being well. She had been on a 40-week agricultural course that required 70–80 hour working weeks of hard physical labor. At the end of the year she had all the symptoms back plus tonsillitis that was not improved by more than three weeks of gradually increasing antibiotics and immense fatigue. All the medical tests were negative. The only thing that worked, was rest and six weeks of all the best self-management techniques she knew before she was 80% recovered and then a few months more of 'more rest than usual' before she could go into the work force.

Stage five: no recovery and cases of 'always been ill'

One of the more difficult situations for the physician to have to manage is a patient who is both chronically and severely ill and for whom medical interventions give little relief. The important issue is never to give up hope. One of us (HDP) had CFS for 34 years and recovered in six weeks, with no relapses in the 15 years since. As her doctor, JCM had been very concerned about the apparent hopelessness of the case. Fortunately, he had managed to convey otherwise and to project at least some faith and hope for a more positive future. This was part of what made it possible for HDP to take the steps that lead to remission and recovery.

Another group who are 'difficult' are those who do not quite fit the CFS criteria because they have 'always been ill'. While researchers like to describe people who had a clear-cut entry to the ill state, some physicians are going to have patients who have all the symptoms and cannot remember never having them. Formal research and diagnostic categories require that these people not be included as a 'true CFS' case. However, this does not mean these people do not exist. They do and they, too, need a diagnosis and committed care that begins right now.

Immediate care and all the management issues are the same for both the cases of 'no recovery' and those who cannot remember when they became ill as for those who are in the chronic stages of the illness.

Coping strategies

The coping strategies of those with CFS in this stage seem to be heterogeneous with some being able to accept the difficult symptoms and others who seek to expend their energy traveling around the country and the world looking for an explanation and some relief from their suffering.

In a study of the patients' view of CFS (Murdoch, 1995), cluster analysis identified four groups of people, two of which improved and two who did less well. The most improved group (91% female) had a low rate of referral to specialists, a low use of antidepressants and tranquilizers and a low use of complementary treatments. The group who did worst of all had tried four times as many treatments, including alternative therapies, had seen five times as many professionals, had a high rate of antidepressant and tranquilizer use, and a high rate of referral to psychiatrists. The important issue is the fact that these clusters seemed to respond to the problem in quite different ways. We are not claiming that there was a causal relationship between seeking help and getting worse; perhaps they sought alternative therapists and psychiatrists because they were worse. However, it is interesting that those people who saw the least number of professionals and tried the least number of treatments seemed to do best.

The heterogeneity of this group draws attention to the way people cope with chronic illness. Shapiro (1983) has proposed that most coping strategies may be understood as an attempt to maintain a sense of control over life in general, or over the outcomes of the illness in particular. In this regard, work on locus of control becomes relevant as individuals may maintain a sense of control through a belief in personal efficacy (active participation in the recovery process), through a belief in chance or through a belief in powerful others. Applying this to the coping strategies of families coping with a physically ill or handicapped child, she proposed a four-quadrant model of control which is divided into dimensions of active and passive control, as well as positive and negative control.

	ACTIVE	PASSIVE
POSITIVE	1	2
NEGATIVE	3	4

1 **Active positive.** Information seeking, direction of action regarding the illness, tackling strategies, mastery of specific illness-related strategies, goal setting.

   Gerry was a university professor who became ill after a severe attack of flu in 1982. His main symptoms were extreme fatigue and weakness, chronic abdominal pain, diarrhea, mental confusion, sleep disturbance and severe muscle pains. Things got so bad at one time that he had himself admitted to a psychiatric ward. In spite of his illness he managed to spend much time in the library researching the problem and was instrumental in setting up the local branch of the CFS support group.

2 **Passive positive.** Insight, acceptance, continuing to live life as fully as possible, given the constraints of the illness.

   Tony was a 35-year-old school teacher and counselor who became ill with CFS in 1982. He was so ill he had to go to bed each night straight after school, got up at 8 pm for an hour and then slept all night. His doctor was supportive and told him that more and more people were getting like this and that his symptoms were nothing to worry about. After six months Tony forced him to refer him to a psychiatrist who told Tony he was mentally normal and reacting really positively to a physical illness. Two years on from the start of this illness, Tony said that 'things have quietly improved. Many who have known me right through this period don't even know that I have been ill. I am positive and, in fact, thankful for some of the changes CFS has forced on me.'

3 **Active negative.** Obsessional hypervigilance, dysfunctional denial and avoidance, anger and rejection of the illness.

   Lynley was a 37-year-old self-employed caterer who had been ill for the past six years. Her symptoms improved when she took time off work but she felt unable to take things easy. She came only infrequently to see her usual doctor and when she came it was usually to tell him about some new treatment she was trying such as a candida diet, electroacupuncture, homeopathy, crystals. She would not be seen dead at an CFS support meeting nor would she ever tell anyone that she had the illness.

4 **Passive negative.** Capitulation, focus on helplessness, hopelessness and pervasive dependency, feelings of depression and low self-esteem, resignation and giving up.

> Jean was a 16-year-old shop assistant who became ill with CFS in 1983. She lived at home with her mother and father. Over the three years she became progressively disabled, gave up work and was almost bedridden. Feeling ill continually, she became very depressed and wandered away from home. She was lost in the hills above her home town for 36 hours and was eventually found suffering from exposure. Among the reasons she gave for her depression were frustration and impatience at not being able to get on with her life and the uncertainty and fear of the illness's next move.

It has been interesting to try to relate these models to the people with CFS and to speculate that difference in coping styles might account for the difference in the way people react to their illness. It would seem that the group who did better might approximate most closely to the passive-positive and those who did worst to the active-negative grouping. Focus by the physician in identifying and strengthening coping strategies may therefore be helpful in achieving a better outcome for those in this chronic stage.

Stages in the lifecycle

One of the special characteristics of CFS is its tendency to affect people at all stages of the lifecycle. The most recent prevalence study (Jason *et al.*, 1999) found that the highest prevalence was in the 40–49 age group. In New Zealand the mean age of onset was 28.9 years in women and 30.73 years in men but the difference was not significant. The most common decades of onset were the second, third and fourth decades. It was relatively uncommon to develop the illness before the age of 10 (1%) and after the age of 50 (5%).

When the patient is a child

The diagnosis of any chronic illness in a child is a difficult task in family practice. This can be illustrated by a recent case seen in family practice.

Byron, a previously healthy 10-year-old, presented with a two-month history of fatigue, sore throat and tender glands in the neck, and recurring abdominal pain. Blood tests revealed a high ESR and C-reactive protein but the Paul Bunnel test and Epstein–Barr virology was negative. Although his doctor (JCM) considered CFS as a possibility, he had never seen a case with a high ESR and Byron was referred to a pediatrician who expressed surprise at the referral from a so-called expert in CFS. Further investigations were negative but four weeks later he presented with a perianal abscess. Further investigations revealed that he had multiple abscesses in the small bowel and that the diagnosis was Crohn's disease.

The New Zealand experience is that CFS in a child aged less than 10 years is rare and that other diagnoses should be vigorously sought before labeling. Bell *et al.* (1991) found a prevalence of 230/100 000 in New York State. Since children aged 10 and under account for approximately 15% of the population in family practice, the chances of a presentation to the physician resulting in this diagnosis are extremely low. However, the problem does occur and CFS was found to be the single most common cause of long-term absence from school in the UK (Dowsett and Colby 1997). The prognosis in children is generally good (Krilov *et al.*, 1998) and it is, therefore, important to manage the illness in a family context, involving the child and the parents at every stage and giving support and education. Liaison with schools will be important, ensuring that the optimal amount of educational and sporting activity is engaged in. As in other presentations of CFS there will undoubtedly be delay and conflict concerning the diagnosis and this is bound to have an effect on the parents and other children. Often, the support of the family doctor will be recruited on one side or other of this conflict and the strength of the doctor–family relationship will be fully tested as will the relationship between the partners in the family. Many pediatricians see themselves as serving in the child's interest where there is a conflict of beliefs about diagnosis and treatment and the family doctor may find him or herself in a difficult position. The important issue is to make the diagnosis according to the criteria and to support both the child and the family in the best possible way.

The issue of control is one of importance in any case of chronic childhood illness. There are occasions when adults must make decisions for the best care of their child but there are probably many more when it is more helpful if the child makes the decisions or at least has some input into the decision-making process. At times of severe illness, options are constrained, but most of the time in CFS in children the questions are of a very practical nature. Should we send him/her to school today? Should we make them eat what is put in front of them? How do we cope on sports day when the school insists that all take part and the child is in remission this week?

The following are some rough rules of thumb for parents making decisions about the care of a child who is not depressed.

- Assume the child will go to school and activities unless there is evidence to the contrary. Consider attending $\frac{1}{2}$ or $\frac{1}{4}$ days at a time. Social relationships are of considerable importance.
- Only the child knows the level of fatigue, pain and other symptoms. Only they can say if and when they can cope at school and socially.
- Set standards of behavior and expectations of self-care (e.g. hygiene) and contribution to the family (e.g. doing the dishes). Self-care and contribution expectations may have to be modified in the light of their symptom levels. Behavior is less modified (e.g. screaming temper tantrums should only be in the time-out room, not in the family room in front of visitors).
- Make a safe place where the child can feel good about themselves, even when the symptom levels are high and they feel irritable.
- When children are given the freedom and responsibility for making decisions they sometimes make the wrong ones or the outcomes might be unpredictable. While keeping to certain standards of behavior, support them as they learn about cause and effect. Allow them time to recover if they overdo it.
- Allow some risk-taking both in relation to activities that may increase their symptom levels and also in relation to social and physical activities. The latter increases their skill levels, the former will be necessary during their recovery stage when you want them to step out and do more.

Schools have a tendency to be authoritarian and the expectation for school attendance can become one of compulsion. There are also some teachers, psychologists and doctors who would wish to label a child's fatigue and irritability as 'school phobia' and deal with it by insisting on school attendance as if that will deal with the symptoms. If attendance at school stops the symptoms then the child does not have CFS. Parents may need a clinician's support as they relate to such a school and attempt to modify the school's expectations.

It is recognized that high stress is a contributing factor to exacerbations in CFS. Where the school environment is very stressful due to standards that are impossible to meet or such problems as bullying or an overbearing teacher, the child may develop high levels of symptoms during the school hours but have far fewer and more manageable symptoms outside of school. This is not a problem of the child but of the school and alternatives should be explored.

When the patient is an adolescent

The management of the person between 11 and 20 years is said to be difficult in family practice, although a New Zealand study (Murdoch and Silva, 1996) of the views of 861 18-year-olds found both high usage and high satisfaction. The same project also looked at the prevalence of disability and found that 160 per 1000 had some disability in endurance (sitting, standing and exercises), suggesting that problems of fatigue are common in the adolescent (Langley et al., 1995).

Often, the management of adolescents is very difficult because the patient is dragged along as an unwilling subject for diagnosis by overanxious parents.

> Robert, aged 16, was brought to the doctor by his mother who had suffered from CFS for many years. An older sister was also known to have CFS. Robert was causing havoc at home, fighting with his father because of his smoking, under-age drinking and staying out late with his friends. His mother asked the doctor to examine him to see if he had CFS as she felt that he was unwell.

In this case it would have been all too easy for the doctor to assume that the mother was presenting somatic symptoms on behalf of her beloved son to protect him from the wrath of his father and to cover up emotional and developmental problems. However, an objective appraisal including talking to Robert alone, examining him thoroughly and doing appropriate investigations including those for EBV revealed that he had the criteria for CFS.

The vital issue in the approach to the adolescent is the offering of an independent, personal and confidential service to them as individuals. The development of symptoms such as fatigue, pain, headache, sleep disturbance and memory loss can be a devastating blow to the confidence and stability of the adolescent. It is interesting to reflect on the extent to which moderate to severe acne vulgaris can devastate teenagers and to understand how much more CFS can affect them. Chronic illness in this age group can have serious consequences such as suicide, co-existent depression and eating disorders, and their onset can be easily missed. On the other hand, a too-facile acceptance of an apparently simple diagnosis such as CFS can allow families to conceal other difficulties long enough for them to become chronic. A recent study (Garralda et al., 1999) has shown that, even after recovery from CFS, there is an increased risk of psychiatric disorder, as anxiety disorders were significantly more common in recovered subjects than in those with active CFS illness status.

The most important risk faced by adolescents with CFS is suicide. In 1986, after an article about CFS in the media, JCM received this letter.

> Dear Professor,
> I enclose a cheque for $100 which I hope can be used for your research into ME. I read all about this in the article in *The Listener* last week. My son Gerald went to our GP about six weeks ago complaining of symptoms which were identical to those described in your article. The doctor got very upset with Gerald and told him to 'go and get a life'. That weekend Gerald took his own life.

The money was collected at his funeral service and we were wondering what to do with it. Having read what you said, I think Gerald had ME and I hope that the money can be used to help educate doctors so that this kind of thing might not happen again.

Many adolescents with CFS, even before a diagnosis, have died at their own hand because they cannot tolerate the confusion and the suffering that these symptoms bring to them. At the very least we have to offer unconditional immediate care to them so that they can develop the confidence to disclose the feelings and the fears which are giving them so much difficulty.

Important co-morbidities in this age group are depression and eating disorders. Those who believe that food allergies and sensitivities play a role in the management of CFS must ensure that a difficult situation is not made worse by the encouragement of eating disorders. Liaison with specialists in these areas is important, remembering always that there is a continuing role for the family doctor in co-ordinating the care of day to day problems in all members of the family. The tendency to separate specialized services from primary care issues is very often unhelpful to the on-going care of such families.

Dunedin is a major university city in New Zealand and many of the adolescents seen with CFS were in the early years of university. Often, this was their first time away from home and family, and student halls of residence or low-rental apartments are not the optimum places in which to be ill. Further education is supposed to provide the opportunity to think critically and in this, the importance of memory and recall is fundamental, as are self-discipline, self-control and the management of finances. Thus, a whole raft of issues arose from the symptoms of CFS which student health personnel found difficult to manage.

Much of the value of student and adolescent life lies in the area of socializing with groups outside the family and childhood community. In most societies this involves the development of sexuality and the use of alcohol and drugs. Associated with the symptoms of CFS might be sexual difficulties, menstrual worsening and alcohol intolerance, and those who work with adolescents with CFS have to be aware of these and make it clear that they are willing to discuss these and offer help.

When the person is pregnant and/or a mother

Wendy is quite a common example of females in her age group, as many of those affected with CFS are in the child-bearing and rearing years and ask for advice concerning the risk to unborn and present children of the maternal illness. We often meet the problem of the couple who recognize that the wife is too ill to be in paid employment and so they decide to have a baby! In our experience most women with CFS who become pregnant improve. Perhaps it is the 'sick' role awarded to pregnancy which helps, although the main improving factor may be the additional circulation provided by the developing fetus.

The problems tend to reoccur after the birth of the baby when the physical and emotional demands of looking after the newborn and the other children may exacerbate the symptoms. A significant minority of women (7% in our series) first develop CFS at this time, suggesting that such women may be particularly vulnerable. It is also a time when all mothers are susceptible to psychological stress. A prospective study comparing the psychological health of mothers of Down's syndrome children and control children (Murdoch and Ogston, 1984) showed that the same proportion of both groups developed psychological problems in the year following birth. If this can happen to healthy mothers, then it is perhaps not surprising that those with CFS might be vulnerable.

Where the person is in the workforce

Given the long course of the disabling symptoms in CFS it is not surprising that there are reports of difficulties in maintaining employment. Tiredness, co-ordination and difficulty in concentrating have been reported as being a major problem (Murdoch and Bradshaw, 1984). In the Chicago prevalence study (Jason et al., 1999), individuals with CFS were more likely to be receiving disability income, working part-time or be unemployed than were controls.

Thus, a major topic at an early stage after making the diagnosis will be managing work with the relapsing illness and dealing with concentration problems, particularly in occupations such as driving, operating heavy machinery and flying. There will also be resulting financial and morale concerns if paid work is limited or not possible. In certain cultures these will affect males more and breadwinner issues will be important. There will also be problems in certain countries in meeting medical bills or in losing employment-related health benefits. It is interesting that only 50% of the Chicago CFS patients had a physician overseeing the disease and costs must be a major factor in this.

Where the person with chronic fatigue syndrome is older

The older a person becomes, the more symptoms they develop, and the more difficult it is to diagnose CFS with certainty. Of the 412 people seen in Dunedin, only one was over the age of 60 when she developed the problem and the trigger was EBV with positive laboratory testing. In medicine there is a saying, *Never say never*, and the elderly can develop the symptoms just like anyone else. However, the range of illnesses associated with fatigue, headache, muscle pain, cognitive deficit, memory loss, sleep disturbance is so much greater in the elderly and the doctor has often to be much more vigilant about the diagnosis. Perhaps the main reason why the elderly are seldom diagnosed as having CFS is that the stringent conditions for obtaining the sick role are relaxed as we get older and the expectations of individuals are much less.

Conclusion

CFS has been described as an *equal-opportunity disorder*. Although we know that it is more likely to affect young women in the child-bearing age, like Wendy, it can strike anyone at any time. Therefore, the number of permutations and combinations on the theme of the illness of CFS is endless. For this reason it is hard from the viewpoint of the family or the family doctor to understand the abstractions of writers who portray the suffering of the typical CFS person as being:

> exacerbated by a self-perpetuating, self-validating cycle in which common, endemic, somatic symptoms are incorrectly attributed to serious abnormality, reinforcing the patient's belief that he or she has a serious disease. (Barsky and Borus, 1999)

Applied to our patient Wendy, this abstraction seems fatuous because her disease has never been recognized, let alone used for any purpose. One of the differences about the family practitioner, according to McWhinney (1996), is that we tend to think in terms of individual patients rather than generalized abstractions. While this may be the opposite end of a spectrum it is difficult to understand the possible value of abstractions which portray people with *functional somatic syndromes* so negatively. If they are *characterized more by symptoms, suffering and disability than by consistently demonstrable tissue abnormality*, then the way forward is individual care with particular emphasis on understanding the whole person and helping to prevent further disability. As will be explained in the next chapter, professionals need no encouragement to devalue the lives of those with chronic illness, particularly where there is no demonstrable tissue abnormality.

> The closer we are, the fuller our knowledge of particulars. The greater the distance, the greater the degree of abstraction. (McWhinney, 1996)

As we have already said in Chapter 1, each family doctor may well have only one person with CFS for whom they can provide care at any time in the lifecycle.

If there are maladaptive responses with functional or dysfunctional patterns of behavior, there is much more chance of these being dealt with at an individual and family level by a doctor who is committed to a relationship with the person and the family unit.

References

Barsky AJ and Borus JF (1999) Functional somatic syndromes: a review. *Ann Intern Med.* 130: 910–21.

Bell KM, Cookfair D, Bell DS, Reese P and Cooper L (1991) Risk factors associated with chronic fatigue syndrome in a cluster of pediatric cases. *Rev Infect Dis.* 13 (Suppl 1): S32–S38.

Cassell E (1991) *The Nature of Suffering and the Goals of Medicine.* Oxford University Press, Oxford, UK.

Dowsett EG and Colby J (1997) Long-term sickness absence due to ME/CFS in UK schools: an epidemiological study with medical and educational implications. *J Chronic Fatigue Synd.* 3: 29–42.

Garralda E, Rangel L, Levin M and Roberts H (1999) Psychiatric adjustment in adolescents with a history of chronic fatigue syndrome. *J Am Acad Child Adolesc Psychiatry.* 38: 1515–21.

Jason LA, Richman JA, Rademaker AW et al. (1999) A community based study of chronic fatigue syndrome. *Arch Intern Med.* 159: 2129–37.

Krilov LR, Fisher M, Friedman SB, Reitman D and Mandel FS (1998) Course and outcome of chronic fatigue in children and adolescents. *Pediatrics.* 102: 360–6.

Langley JD, Stanton WR, McGee R and Murdoch JC (1995) Disability in late adolescence I. Introduction, methods and overview. *Disabil Rehabil.* 17: 35–42.

McKinley RK and Middleton JF (1999) What do patients want from doctors? Content analysis of written patient agendas for the consultation. *Br J Gen Pract.* 49: 796–800.

McWhinney IR (1989) 'An acquaintance with particulars...'. *Fam Med.* 21: 296–8.

McWhinney IR (1996) The importance of being different. *Br J Gen Pract.* 46: 433–6.

Murdoch JC (1995) *Chronic fatigue syndrome: the patient-centered view.* Proceedings of 'ME: the patient oriented approach' conference, 10–12 February, Dunedin, New Zealand.

Murdoch JC and Bradshaw PW (1984) Mystery illness in Dunedin. In: JC Murdoch (Chair), *The ME syndrome: a one day seminar.* 17 November, University of Otago, New Zealand.

Murdoch JC and Ogston SA (1984) Down's syndrome children and parental psychological upset. *J R Coll Gen Pract.* 34: 87–90.

Murdoch JC and Silva PA (1996) The use of general practitioner services by eighteen-year-olds in New Zealand. *NZ Med J.* 109: 113–15.

Shapiro J (1983) Family reactions and coping strategies in response to the physically ill or handicapped child: a review. *Soc Sci Med.* 17: 913–31.

Stephens GG (1982) *The intellectual basis of family practice.* Winter Publishing Company, Tucson, AZ.

Stewart M, Brown JB, Weston WW *et al.* (1995) *Patient-Centered Medicine: transforming the clinical method.* Sage Publications, Thousand Oaks, CA.

5

Mad, bad or dangerous to know? The societal context of chronic fatigue syndrome

Case study
Wendy's problems just do not seem to go away. One morning the symptoms are worse than ever and just to complicate matters, Willie's mother Gladys calls for a visit. She is appalled at the state of the house and the children and, after leaving, contacts Wendy's parents so that together they can try to 'help' Wendy. Gladys goes to see Dr Rose for her three-monthly check and can't help mentioning to him that she is worried about the family. Dr Rose tells her in no uncertain terms that he knows Wendy needs help but that she refuses to listen to him.

Gladys phones Willie and tells him all this and suggests that he goes along with his father-in-law's kind offer to send Wendy to LA. She will look after him and the children and Wendy can go for 'as long as it takes.' Willie loses his temper and tells her to mind her own business and that he and Wendy can sort out their own affairs. Gladys then gets in touch with Wendy's parents and they agree that both Willie and Wendy were 'being difficult' and 'obviously didn't want anyone to help'. 'They would be left to work things out for themselves!'

Wendy feels that her main requirement is for help with the childcare and housework and contacts Social Services for some assistance. The social worker there visits her and asks for permission to approach Dr Rose to verify her diagnosis and get a recommendation. She phones back a week later to say that, having discussed things with the doctor, 'it seems to be a mental health matter', and that she can only get help if she agrees to be seen by a psychiatrist. Wendy becomes very aggressive on the phone and tells the lady that she wishes to have nothing more to do with her.

'Society' as described in this case study has many faces. The institutions represented are families and friends, the health sector, the employment sectors, and the financial sector. The person with the illness can no longer fulfill her expected roles as mother, wife, daughter, daughter-in-law, financial advisor and all the other players have to decide whether her withdrawal is justified or not. The stress of the relationship difficulties converts the other members of the family into potential patients and blame and guilt causes additional problems. The suffering for Wendy has been immense but if she had been found to have terminal cancer, almost certainly the response would have been quite different. Because of the validity of that diagnosis and the sympathy that it evokes in society, she and her husband would have been totally absolved from all responsibilities. Even long-standing family feuds might be settled by the diagnosis and its implications. However, for Wendy, the situation seems to go from bad to worse and the extended family gets in on the act with the final result that even the helping agencies are caught up in the emotional trauma. The key issue seems to be that Dr Rose is confirmed in his explanatory model of Wendy's illness which is that she has a psychiatric disorder. Her entry to help with the house and the children is through an interview with a psychiatrist and this makes her so angry that she cuts herself off from her sources of help.

This case study is very typical of the conflicts produced by this illness and in this chapter we will try to describe and explain why there is such a problem with Wendy and people like her having CFS. The question is a very complex one and the most we can hope for is to give some insights into the enormity of the difficulties faced. The central problem is that there are two contrasting conceptions developed by society to explain why people like Wendy become sick. The first is that she has become disabled because of the unremitting nature of her symptoms and that she requires help from various agencies to help her through the difficulties of her illness. The second is that she has some inherent non-remedial (and punishable) personality problem that drives her to extract sympathy from others by having the symptoms. These, of course, are the extreme views and most people would hold a position that is some point along the line between. According to the one extreme, what Parsons (1975) has called the incapacity model, she has failed in her attempts to remain well as a mother and so the illness allows her to consult a doctor who pronounces her sick, gives her the sick role and society then helps her and the family to get better through medical treatment and social support. According to the other extreme, the deviancy model, illness is a device whereby Wendy can take advantage of it to punish her husband and the other members of the family and milk the benefits of the health and disability agencies.

For all individuals affected by illness there is an impression gained about the relative importance of these two extremes. Illness can elevate some people almost to sainthood and others can be regarded as a figure of fun or a confidence trickster. For many years, people with CFS have had problems because society, in all the forms described above, has tended to decide that they are people 'who enjoy poor health', and who are not to be taken very seriously. Everywhere there has been a problem with CFS, the health professionals and the media have given out subtle and not so subtle messages that somehow these people are fraudulently trying to rip off the health system. Headlines such as 'Scientists prove that shirkers are really sick', and the use of descriptions such as 'yuppie flu' or somatization disorder send out a clear message.

A major problem is that fatigue is a universal symptom, and the use of the term CFS fails completely to convey the full meaning of its whole range of symptoms and disabilities. ME was an incorrect term but at least it had the advantage of conveying the sense of a serious disorder. The Oxford Dictionary gives the meaning of fatigue as 'extreme tiredness after exertion'. However, most of the people with CFS have extreme tiredness without exertion, and indeed the fatigue they have is the very least of their problems. The frightening 'crash', the fact that disabling symptoms last for years, the violent headaches, muscle pain, sleep disturbance, memory loss are all violently painful experiences. Anyone who has listened to these agonizing stories knows that this is far from being a benign condition and that it is not the sort of scenario that shirkers would adopt. Even without the problem of being considered deviant there are difficulties in interacting with others.

A second problem is that some doctors are unwilling to give the sick role unless there is some good evidence of physical illness. For them, subjective evidence is not good enough and they therefore describe CFS and similar illnesses as functional somatic syndromes.

> This term has been applied to several related syndromes characterized more by symptoms, suffering, and disability than by consistently demonstrable tissue abnormality. (Barsky and Borus, 1999)

The list of illnesses described under this banner makes intriguing reading because there are broadly two groups. The first group include health problems which have given governments and insurers great difficulty through various forms of litigation, e.g. the sick building syndrome, repetitive strain injury, the side effects of silicone breast implants, the Gulf War syndrome and chronic whiplash. The second group contains three illnesses where sufferers have had continued symptoms without pathological confirmation, and these are irritable bowel syndrome, fibromyalgia and CFS. Interestingly, exempt from discussion are the psychological disorders that certainly have no demonstrable tissue abnormality.

So Wendy and those like her may leave the doctor's room without the sick role and this leads to many problems both within her family and the community and with the health system in general.

Problems within the family and community

For the person with CFS, taking part in community activities is a very big problem. The relapsing nature of the condition means that responsibilities accepted in good faith while well can often not be fulfilled when a relapse occurs. If this is a one-off occasion allowances are made without too much problem, but second and subsequent lapses in not meeting societal commitments are not well received. This can be particularly difficult for those who are used to being stalwarts of the local community.

> Quiet, self-effacing but highly productive Marion was secretary of her school committee, the most effective member of the swimming club fundraising group and a volunteer for the local blind community. When she became ill for the first time the groups she was in marked time, waiting for her recovery. When she became well enough to manage attending the meetings she found very little had been done and people were waiting for her to organize them again. Weighed down with their expectations and the accumulated tasks she struggled to manage while still not very well. Within a month she had a serious relapse, becoming confined initially to bed and then to her house. The groups she was involved in reacted differently. One simply replaced her, a second went into recess and the third had members who became very angry, with some members who took her inability to function as before as a personal attack. Several members of this group started some vicious rumors that were still affecting Marion some years later.

Simple forgetfulness that comes with CFS can also be a very real problem. Some find that they forget to undertake a task but because they did not write it down at the time they had no aid to memory and the task only came to mind when someone asked them if they had performed it.

> On one occasion, Joyce got herself ready to go out to the cinema with friends. When she was sitting in the car, getting ready to drive, she found herself wondering where she was going. So she just went back inside, reckoning that if it was important it would come to mind again. It did not and she missed out on an evening she would have enjoyed and her friends did not invite her the next time they organized a similar evening.

> Keith had been unable to work for four years. In an effort to expand his mind and get himself back into the mainstream community he decided to undertake one course at university. He chose geology, as rocks and fossils had been a passion for many years. With his good general knowledge he did

well in the practical work and he found the theory to be interesting. At the end of year exams he went into a relapse and his mind became a complete blank when he had the examination paper in front of him. He was acutely embarrassed by this, not knowing that this was a symptom of his condition. Fortunately, he consulted his medical practitioner about his other symptoms and a medical certificate was provided which enabled Keith to sit special examinations. This time he passed with a respectable mark.

Julie was a middle-ability student who had a satisfactory record at university. At the end of her second year of university she became very ill and developed CFS. During this time, Julie had a reasonable relationship with a doctor who accepted the reality of her condition. After two years she had improved considerably but did not know if she could cope with a full-time course. She consulted her family physician and together they decided that part-time attendance would be better in the first instance. Much to Julie's distress she found that she had lost her ability to think critically. She was unable to access necessary information from books. She could not hold sufficient pieces of information in her mind to make the connections expected in her subject. The end of year examination was a nightmare and Julie only just passed. The university took the stand that academic standards could not be relaxed although they did make some allowances for Julie's relapses, giving her an extension of time. During that year Julie relapsed on two occasions and on both she required a medical certificate to justify not meeting course requirements. She was so upset by the situation that she had not finished her degree at the time of writing.

A more positive story came from the first self-management course held by one of the authors (HDP).

A young woman, engaged to be married, just coped holding down full-time work while sleeping between 12–14 hours a day and most of the weekend. She was worried that she could not manage the wedding both families were planning. Even the weekend trip to the next city to plan the wedding was a major problem. She planned that weekend trip as meticulously as she could, given her 'brain fog', with lists and timelines. On her arrival back she looked radiant. She told me both families had realized that the planned wedding was beyond her, and there was no reason why the couple could not marry immediately. So, with both families present they used the time booked with the priest to get married instead of planning for the big day. Everyone was delighted and a number of small more manageable celebrations were planned for the different groups of relations and social networks. This was the first time I saw her reasonably well and I am sure the love and caring from her husband and both families contributed to her recovery over the next three months.

Katy, a mother of three children managed to appear to cope under most circumstances through careful self- and family management. Her husband Kenny was unsupportive and demanding but as long as there was no additional stress, things looked satisfactory to those outside the family unit. Problems occurred when Kenny announced that he had invited his brother, wife and two young children from overseas to visit for three weeks. When Katy put her foot down and said no, she was not well enough, his response was that either she left home that night and he would get a housekeeper to cook and clean, or she could stay and do it herself.

Steven, 27, had a diagnosis of CFS from his sympathetic family physician. Forms for a sickness benefit were filled in and returned to the government pension office. However, the conditions for benefits had been tightened and the government had decreed that too many people had been put on such benefits. Steven was required to attend a designated doctor who, after a 10-minute interview asking leading questions and not appearing to listen to the answers, said that there was nothing wrong with Steven that a job would not fix. He was then required to attend the employment office for an assessment for work. Steven was very worried as there was no way he could manage to work full time.

So why is it that the impression of CFS as an enjoyable but deviant pastime has arisen? 'Pastime' is perhaps an appropriate term since in the people seen in most series, the time passed between onset and diagnosis is three years or more. Denial of the seriousness of the syndrome takes place at all levels and is difficult for those affected to counter, given the fact that the evidence for their suffering is often entirely subjective.

Problems with the medical system

As has been illustrated by the stories, many doctors are supportive to the people who have CFS, often more out of commitment to individuals and families than by any particular belief in a diagnosis. This knowledge of the family or the individuals allows them to confer the 'sick role' and this helps the person to convince the family and the health and social services to give maximum help in overcoming the disability. A major advantage of this step is to help get the other players to back off for a while and give the person a little room. In Wendy's case, however, there is a different outcome. The doctor cannot recognize the problem, the tests are all normal, she does not need any further tests, or hospitalization. In fact, he wants her to see a psychiatrist and that, for most of society, is a diagnosis and not a suggestion. She returns from her visits to the gatekeeper to the medical system without any ticket of entry to its benefits.

A study of the views of people with CFS in New Zealand (Murdoch, 1995) indicated that virtually all consulted a family physician for their illness and a third found that their family physician was unhelpful or very unhelpful to them in managing the illness. Other studies have found that some general practitioners do not accept the validity of the diagnosis of CFS (Denz-Penhey and Murdoch, 1993; Ho-Yen and Macnamara, 1991). A small Australian study (Woodward *et al.*, 1995) of 20 physicians found that 70% were reluctant to articulate a diagnosis of CFS. They felt constrained by the scientific uncertainty regarding its etiology and by a concern that diagnosis might become a disabling self-fulfilling prophecy.

So, there is a double problem here. It is clear that patients should not diagnose themselves, but where else do they go if their medical advisor either refuses to diagnose or gives them one with which they cannot agree? A case study in the UK suggested that physicians believed that patients who self-diagnosed with CFS were less likely to comply with treatment, more likely to pose difficult management problems and more likely to take up a lot of time (Scott *et al.*, 1995). The authors considered that doctors should remind themselves that their observed attitudes could lead to unsatisfactory consultations, resentment and unnecessarily prolonged disability. This resentment by doctors of people suggesting their own diagnosis has been underlined by Finestone (1997) who comments:

> In my experience with several of these cases, the claimants are highly intelligent with graduate degrees and sophisticated occupations. They all had significant knowledge of CFS, and a coterie of physicians has developed who tout high doses of vitamins, immune-enhancing programs or antibiotic treatments. Some claimants have established a cottage industry for this syndrome.

Here there is no need to rehearse the arguments for and against the balance of power in the patient–doctor relationship. The answer to the question depends on whether you are the doctor or the patient. It is enough to state that the person with CFS was unlikely to be granted the sick role by the average doctor in the year 2000 without a fair degree of difficulty. Perhaps this explains why 50% of the CFS patients in the recent Chicago study (Jason *et al.*, 1999) had not consulted a doctor and why an increasing number seek help from alternative medicine.

At the very least, doctors should be able to treat the people with these symptoms with civility and good manners but this is not always the case. CFS patients are sometimes treated as if they had been caught trying to trick their doctors into giving the sick role. The language in many books and papers on the illness often betrays an adversarial attitude towards any who dare to challenge the current consensus or who have symptoms which do not accord with existing diagnoses. Thus, statements are produced in the scientific literature such as:

the more convinced patients with functional somatic syndromes are that their symptoms are serious and pathologic, the more intense, prolonged, and disabling the symptoms become. Such symptom amplification is fostered by physicians who prematurely focus exclusively on medical explanations for the symptoms, by alarming anecdotes in the popular press and on the internet and by organized campaigns to designate a particular syndrome as a serious disease. (Barsky and Borus, 1999)

This rejection of the good motives of any who dare claim that they have a physical illness is paradoxical, given that it is the medical profession which has stimulated an appetite for procedures and diagnoses in the first place by insisting on consistently demonstrable tissue abnormality (Barsky and Borus, 1999). The patient who will not accept the assurance of professionals that there is nothing wrong with her or him is then a problem to the doctors who insist on control and obedience. It is this attitude and not the difficult-to-understand illness that has given rise to the rudeness and lack of civility that often marks such consultations. The use of terms such as CRUD (chronic relapsing undiagnosable disease) and GOMER (Get Out of My Emergency Room), even the milder 'heartsink' betray a doctor-centered insistence on control. Such physicians often defend their position by accusing patients of fraud and deception, and thus, not surprisingly, stimulating an equal and opposite reaction.

The use and misuse of diagnosis

At the beginning of the new millennium there is a crisis in medicine, and that is that patients are now refusing to accept the decision of doctors as final, much in the same way as Wendy refused to accept that she had a psychiatric disorder. The reason for this refusal seems quite simple, and is that she is not treated respectfully and professionally. She is not stupid and knows perfectly well what Dr Rose is trying to do. He is trying to control her by labeling her with a pseudo-psychological diagnosis with the help of a referral to a psychiatrist. There is nothing particularly sinister about doing that but there is a problem with doing it without her consent. The problem with the current systems of diagnosis for those whose symptoms do not obviously fit into familiar diagnoses is that it is entirely doctor-centered. A group of experts devise criteria for CFS (Holmes et al., 1988) into which she fits and then along come Barsky and Borus (1999) arbitrarily placing CFS in a category entitled 'functional somatic syndromes'. The problem with this diagnosis is that it is not done with a view to treatment but is done distantly without regard either to Wendy or her doctor and usually funded by some government agency. Governments are extremely interested in these classifications for a very good reason: they are an important weapon in the social control of populations, particularly with regard to healthcare expenditure. Most of the experts who discuss these problems are unhindered by any personal experience of dealing with patients with the problem.

CFS has proven to be a very difficult problem, particularly in the US where there are estimated to be 800 000 sufferers. In the UK there has also been strong lobbying from thousands of people affected by the disorder. One of the responses by the medical authorities in both countries has been to attempt to explain the condition as a psychological disorder. Because any physical, psychiatric or addictive disorder has been excluded through the definition, it has been necessary to use terms such has 'somatization disorder' to explain the illness.

It is obvious from the very complicated criteria of somatization disorder (American Psychiatric Association, 1994), that it would take five years of argument by learned counsel before a panel of judges to get a verdict one way or the other. However, in real life the verdict lies in the remit of the likes of Dr Rose, and those who are in favor of this diagnosis are continually pleading for the criteria to be simplified. Kroenke *et al.* (1997) suggest the term 'multisomatoform disorder', defined as three or more current somatoform symptoms from a 15-symptom checklist which have been present for at least two years. At least they have made an attempt to evaluate the outcome of such a classification. Others simply invent their own. The condition of 'somatized mental disorder' (Morriss *et al.*, 1999) has the criteria of :

- a physical complaint lasting for **more than two weeks** where the patient believes complaint has a physical cause
- GHQ-12 score is >3
- family physician does not have evidence from examination or investigations that the patient has a physical pathology that explains all symptoms and disability.

It is important to understand the world view that is driving this approach because only then can justice be done in the consultation. The authors of this article state that:

> one-third of patients with mental disorders in primary care present with physical symptoms that they believe have a physical cause. They have **potentially treatable** psychiatric disorders that cause, exacerbate or maintain the physical symptom or related disability. These patients are said to have somatized mental disorders.

So, at a stroke the definition is modified so that it will be easier for physicians to give an authoritative diagnosis. Note that these problems are only potentially treatable and we will review the evidence for this in Chapter 7. This claim would be legitimate if it had been proven that by giving such a diagnosis the people affected would then have a potentially treatable condition, but there is no evidence that somatized psychiatric disorder is any more or less treatable than CFS.

So where does CFS lie within this spectrum of disorders? The lead author in this research is Goldberg and in a previous review of CFS (Woods and Goldberg, 1991) he concludes:

> The disorder is kept going by disease conviction, by maladaptive beliefs about possibilities of improvement, and by abnormal illness behavior in that exercise is avoided and the patient becomes detrained. There may also be other secondary gains of the sick role in individual cases.

This opinion is shared by many of the psychiatric researchers into CFS (*see* the section on cognitive behavioral therapy in Chapter 7) but seldom is shared face to face with people like Wendy in order to gain their consent. This psychological labeling of people by doctors has caused great distress amongst the many thousands of people who believe that they have CFS.

The major problem with the doctor-centered approach to labeling is that it seems to miss the point that 'patients with persistent somatic symptoms feel blamed, coerced, devalued and misunderstood by any psychological inquiry' (Epstein *et al.*, 1999). This was borne out in the questionnaire study (Murdoch, 1995) where psychiatrists were felt to be the least useful of all practitioners consulted (*see* Chapter 7). Woods and Goldberg (1991) attribute this to a mind–body dualism.

> The sufferers are trapped in the same either/or thinking that has entrapped the medical profession: any doubt cast by a doctor that one's symptoms are entirely physical in origin implies that they are entirely psychological and that is not acceptable.

However, what Woods and Goldberg fail to recognize is that decisions about diagnosis or management in any illness have to be made with the consent of the patient. The discomfort which people with CFS have about being labeled as somatizers or neurasthenics is a reality and it will not be dispelled by capitulation to the labels which have been devised by psychiatrists. Neither is there any evidence that the symptoms resolve with an acceptance of the diagnostic term.

War by media

The frustrations caused by this long-standing suffering and disability inevitably lead to abnormal illness behavior by patients and abnormal treatment behavior by doctors. We only have to observe the pressures set up in the Jones household and the Rose office to understand how these can arise. Since CFS patients are human, there are inevitably some highly disturbed people amongst them. If there are, say, 800 000 people with CFS in the US, it would not be surprising if one or two thousand were trying to draw the attention of their doctors by engaging in some very manipulative behaviors. However, that should not prevent good care from being offered to them or to others who are not manipulative attention-seekers. On the other hand, there are doctors who engage in manipulative behaviors and who use their power to deny the best management to those who need it.

On both the consumer and the medical side, some influential people have become involved and those affected by the illness and infuriated by the reaction of doctors have set up powerful patient groups to challenge and stimulate the equally powerful medical and research lobbies. At first, there seemed to be a sympathetic and co-operative partnership as the doctors and academics did the research which was to authenticate the experience of the patients. However, these happy days were always doomed to pass because neither side seemed to understand where the other was coming from. For the researchers results had to be positive within the pre-existing set of models of a particular discipline for it to be regarded as authentic. What the patients did not realize was that no one can guarantee research results and that research can never authenticate or negate the valid experience of any individual. Almost every parameter, virological, immunological and endocrinological, has been examined either with negative or ambivalent results and the only research findings which seemed to be accepted unreservedly by the medical profession were the observations of the psychiatrists that those who are ill for a long time without a diagnosis are vulnerable to depression, paranoia and really want an organic diagnosis.

Over the last ten years the medical and research lobby has tired of CFS as a research challenge. On the other hand, the CFS lobby groups have been disappointed by the results and have felt betrayed by the willingness of health professionals to accept a psychiatric label which purports to explain the cause for the syndrome. As after a marriage break-up, the arguments on both sides tend to be universal and theoretical and so it has been with the struggle for legitimacy of CFS. The resulting break-up has been bitter and intense. On the one side the proponents of the psychiatric cause seem to have an uncanny knack of amusing their colleagues and upsetting sufferers by rehashing myths about Victorian water and rest cures (Sharpe and Wessely, 1998) and reviving the concept of neurasthenia. Their position is not helped by their association with historians such as Shorter (1992) and Showalter (1997) who openly condemn patients as frauds and label any doctor who is sympathetic to these genuine sufferers as a physician enthusiast. Interestingly, Shorter attributes the epidemic of CFS at the end of the 20th century to two factors: the power of the popular media and the loss of medical authority. Showalter, in her book *Hystories: hysterical epidemics and modern media* (1997), identifies CFS with Gulf War syndrome, recovered memories of sexual abuse, multiple-personality disorder, satanic ritual abuse and alien abduction. She also blames media prompting and therapeutic suggestion for the encouragement of these disorders. One would have thought that such views would be regarded as lunatic fringe, but Shorter was the lead paper in a monograph on CFS produced by the Ciba Foundation in 1993 (Shorter, 1993), and both Shorter and Showalter are, unbelievably, quoted in scientific papers such as that of Barsky and Borus (1999) as scientific evidence for their concerns:

> Physicians in many medical specialties are increasingly confronted by patients who have disabling, medically unexplained somatic symptoms and who have already arrived at a diagnostic label for their illness. The functional somatic syndromes have acquired major sociocultural and political dimensions. Their definitive status in public consciousness and popular discourse contrasts markedly with their still uncertain scientific and biomedical status.

It is difficult for some of us to see the Wendy Joneses of this world in that definition and some of these writers seem inordinately threatened by the power of the lobby for the patients. Indeed, they seem puzzled that CFS sufferers cannot accept the simple solution which is to accept the diagnosis of psychological disorder.

The societal lesson for the large CFS support groups in this media battle has been that it is impossible to assume that the medical academic and research lobby will act in the best interests of the people affected. It is perfectly obvious that many of the estimates of prevalence by doctors were absurdly low and Jason's Chicago study demonstrated that 50% of those affected had not consulted doctors about their problem (Jason *et al.*, 1999). The full-circle return to the explanatory model that CFS is a functional somatic syndrome is unacceptable to the vast majority of sufferers and their doctors and it is astounding that people should be expected to accept such a demeaning explanation.

The surprising issue is that the researchers should expect people to accept the results of their research. Much of the tone of the conclusions of research and review by doctors is authoritarian and seems to demand submission and obedience to psychiatric assessment. Insistence on this approach will lead to a slow decline in the influence of medical research and another institution, more person-centered will rise to take its place. The medical community often fails to realize that times have changed.

> The practice of medicine is being transformed by a powerful set of interlocking trends; evidence-based medicine, clinical governance, consumerism, litigation, resource limitation, devolved budgets and the ending of the profession's monopoly of medical knowledge. (Hodgkin, 2000)

The battle for the intellectual high ground of CFS is being fought in the wrong place. It has to be fought not in the clinics clustering around self-appointed subspecialists, but in the places where people like Wendy meet with people like Dr Alan Rose. People with CFS are increasingly gaining their information from the media and self-help groups rather than from health professionals (Elliot, 1999). This emphasizes the need to build a therapeutic relationship at the interpersonal level between doctor and patient.

The recent history of CFS research demonstrates the limitations of the media, lay and medical circles in providing positive leadership to both patients and doctors. If some as yet unknown virus had been discovered to be the cause for CFS, as happened with Acquired Immune Deficiency Syndrome (AIDS) the researchers would have received all the credit. Now that no such cause has been found with CFS, the sufferers are being given the blame. The medical journals, which insist on scientific accuracy for their research papers, are not so discerning about the generalizing in their editorials and reviews and seem to delight in publishing misleading opinions about sufferers such as have been quoted. No medical problem was ever yet solved by exposure in the media, and none was ever yet solved without full collaboration between doctors and patients.

Trying to find a new way

The end result of the care of Wendy Jones was forcible exclusion from the benefits of care unless she agreed to be seen by a psychiatrist. She was the square peg who could not be fitted into the round hole of an acceptable diagnosis. Her interpretation of that decision is that she is mad, bad or dangerous to know and it therefore became very difficult for her to remain in a good relationship with her doctor.

The main failure of the health system with respect to the management of the person with CFS lies squarely in the inability of medicine in general, and general practice in particular, to honor and cherish the relationship between the persons of the doctor and the patient and to place the needs of persons above the political, economic and technological needs of the health system. At the end of the day it was Wendy's own doctor who let her down. The adoption of a person-centered approach, starting at the initial consultation, could have meant that all those who have the criteria could be healed within that setting. Multiply that failing a million times and you have the vast societal difficulties which are now present. It is difficult to avoid the view that the health system is there for the benefit of its professionals and that those who do not fit the system are either rejected or squeezed into categories which may be inappropriate. Only a return to a realization of the healing power in the patient–doctor relationship will give those with CFS some hope of recovery.

Conclusion

The headlines which have appeared in the press over the past twenty years have told a fascinating story about the way society regards CFS.

> Mystery Disease hits West Otago! ME patients sick of Prejudice! An Illness Doctors don't recognize! Doctors finally prove shirkers are really sick! We were treated as nut cases! The stealthy epidemic of exhaustion!

The editorials in distinguished medical journals have also had interesting titles.

> Royal Free Disease: perplexity continues. Fatigue syndrome: neurasthenia revived. Chronic Fatigue Syndrome: what's in a name? Is it a recognisable disease associated with a unique pathophysiology, or a ragbag of non-specific symptoms with many causes?

The portrayal of the *typical* CFS patient in the general and medical media betrays an underlying desire to deal with a problem which disturbs society. Doctors have always regarded their care as a desirable commodity and have always been suspicious of people who pretend to be ill in order to seek their attention. Part of their professional power and standing lies in their ability to tell whether people are sick or not, and they are pretty sensitive about the fact that deciding on that is sometimes a difficult call. The media love to make a fuss when they get it wrong, either individually or collectively, and the notion that they may be missing a whole new category of disease is a good story. The idea of a rather pompous profession caught with its pants down as the world is secretly attacked by a stealthy epidemic is appealing and amusing to many people who read newspapers. There are those who believe that all this is due to the clever media manipulations of CFS sufferers but that is most unlikely. The main stimulus is the perceived power and privilege of the medical profession which still persists and is even strengthened by the new health reforms which concentrate on controlling the cost of medical treatment.

Having spent the last 50 years encouraging the public to utilize specialist investigations and treatments for every symptom, the medical profession is now faced with a large group of people who are so tired that they cannot function in society. At the same time they are being warned by their masters and funders that resources are limited and that society cannot afford to spend any more money on investigation and treatment. Trying to convince the people with fatigue that they have a psychiatric disorder is one option but, unfortunately, most of the people are unconvinced by that argument.

Some people, including some doctors, may try to pretend that the problems are all being caused by an unruly and rebellious group of people, like Wendy

Jones, who are so sick that they have the time and energy to make trouble in the media. This is a trivial and amusing diversion from the real truth, which is that society needs to be underpinned by care and not investigation and cure, and that unless each family like the Jones has access to person-centered care through a good patient–physician relationship, we are going to be in more and more trouble as the years go on.

References

American Psychiatric Association (1994) *Diagnostic and Statistical Manual of Mental Disorders* (4e). American Psychiatric Association, Washington DC.

Barsky AJ and Borus JF (1999) Functional somatic syndromes: a review. *Ann Intern Med.* **130**: 910–21.

Denz-Penhey H and Murdoch JC (1993) General practitioners' acceptance of the validity of chronic fatigue syndrome as a diagnosis. *NZ Med J.* **106**: 122–4.

Elliot H (1999) Use of formal and informal care among people with prolonged fatigue: a review of the literature. *Br J Gen Pract.* **49**: 131–4.

Epstein RM, Quill TE and McWhinney IR (1999) Somatization reconsidered: incorporating the patient's experience of illness. *Arch Intern Med.* **15**: 215–22.

Finestone AJ (1997) A doctor's dilemma: is a diagnosis disabling or enabling? *Arch Intern Med.* **157**: 491–2.

Ho-Yen DO and McNamara I (1991) General practitioners' experience of the chronic fatigue syndrome. *Br J Gen Pract.* **41**: 324–6.

Hodgkin P (2000) Postcards from a new century. Navigating the new primary care: a pilot. *Br J Gen Pract.* **50**: 78–9.

Holmes GP, Kaplan JE, Gantz N *et al.* (1988) Chronic fatigue syndrome: a working case definition. *Ann Intern Med.* **108**: 387–9.

Jason LA, Richman JA, Rademaker AW *et al.* (1999) A community-based study of chronic fatigue syndrome. *Arch Intern Med.* **159**: 2129–37.

Kroenke K, Spitzer RL, deGruy FV 3rd *et al.* (1997) Multisomatoform disorder. An alternative to undifferentiated somatoform disorder for the somatizing patient in primary care. *Arch Gen Psychiatry.* **54**: 352–8.

Morriss RK, Gask L, Ronalds C *et al.* (1999) Clinical and patient satisfaction outcomes of a new treatment for somatized mental disorder taught to general practitioners. *Br J Gen Pract.* **49**: 263–7.

Murdoch JC (1995) *Chronic fatigue syndrome: the patient-centered view.* Proceedings of 'ME: the patient oriented approach' conference, 10–12 February, Dunedin, New Zealand.

Parsons T (1975) The sick role and the role of the physician reconsidered. *Milbank Mem Fund Q.* **53**: 257–78.

Scott S, Deary I and Pelosi AJ (1995) General practitioners' attitudes to patients with a self-diagnosis of myalgic encephalomyelitis. *BMJ.* **310**: 508.

Sharpe M and Wessely S (1998) Putting the rest cure to rest – again. *BMJ.* **316**: 796.

Shorter E (1992) *From Paralysis to Fatigue: a history of psychosomatic illness in the modern era.* The Free Press, New York.

Shorter E (1993) Chronic fatigue in historical perspective. *Ciba Found Symp.* **173**: 6–16.

Showalter E (1997) *Hystories: hysterical epidemics and modern media.* Columbia University Press, New York.

Woods TO and Goldberg DP (1991) Psychiatric perspectives: an overview. *Br Med Bull.* **47**: 908–18.

Woodward RV, Broom DH and Legge DG (1995) Diagnosis in chronic illness: disabling or enabling: the case of chronic fatigue syndrome. *J R Soc Med.* **88**(6): 325–9.

6

The patient–clinician relationship

Case study
The patient–clinician relationship became increasingly strained as Dr Rose moved from focussing on the cause to possible psychosocial factors that might explain the continuing condition. Wendy felt blamed for her lack of recovery. In addition, her need for symptom control was not being addressed. The doctor's focus on cause and psychosocial factors meant that he was not concerned with the symptoms that brought Wendy to the consultation. The doctor sensed her frustration and growing anger and suggested she return fortnightly for continuing oversight into her condition and so he could reassure her of his concern and continuing care for her as a person. She interpreted this as his using her as a steady stream of income when he was not able to do anything for her. She became so angry at this that she changed doctors.

Testimony of the crisis

One of the major miscalculations which doctors make in dealing with people with CFS is the failure to realize that the central issue in the illness is the crash. The experience of those doctors who have seen many hundreds of people with CFS is that they come to the consultation hurt and confused that family and relatives, workmates and friends and above all their own doctor have failed to appreciate the catastrophic change in their lives caused by this illness. Harvey Cox (1973) has pointed to the importance of testimony in the human experience.

Testimony is me telling my story in a world of people with stories to tell.

People with CFS come to the consultation with their particular story to tell and yet a major difficulty seems to be that no one, not even their doctor, wants to listen. Before they are allowed to talk about what has happened, people, including their doctor, had gone on to other things like wondering what it was, what was the cause and seemed to have switched off into another world.

This takes us back to the classification of Marinker (1983) in dividing patient–doctor interactions into three types, routines, rituals and dramas, and this one is most definitely a drama. This first consultation is the result of a crisis and the major difficulty seems to be that the other participant in the consultation, the doctor, does not seem to realize or agree that a crisis exists.

The management of the crisis and what is done at that point is the issue that we must, therefore, emphasize. There are many similar situations such as the birth of a handicapped child, stillbirth and neo-natal death, the diagnosis of serious illness and lessons should be taken from these to help us in enabling the patient–doctor relationship issues to be improved. For example, in the literature on communicating the diagnosis of a Down's syndrome baby there is clear evidence from mothers of the conditions which they wish to be met by those who are telling them. Mothers wish to be told the diagnosis as quickly as possible after birth, they wish to be told in private with their partner present and they wish to have a supportive and sympathetic general practitioner to help with the considerable problem of caring for a Down's syndrome child. However, when we ask such mothers what happens in real life, we hear some extraordinary stories, such as:

> My GP made it clear that he felt I was being totally selfish by keeping my baby. He said I wasn't considering my 20-month-old son because 'How is he going to feel when he's 15 and bringing his friends home and that blubbering big thing is sitting in the corner?'
>
> My GP is an abrupt man, showing no compassion. The first thing he said was 'I'm sorry about your daughter and if you're thinking about adoption, I think you'll find it hard with a disabled child'. (Murdoch, 1984)

Referring to this communication in a crisis, Franklin (1958) wrote in the language of his time:

> The doctor who tells parents that their baby is a mongol is performing a surgical operation without an anaesthetic; let him be the one who feels deeply about this problem, deeply enough even to pray before the interview and to weep afterwards. But the more deeply he feels, the more need there is for him to have thought deeply, too. Whatever words are spoken, however many the talks, there are two moments in time to be bridged: the last in which the parents look with joy at their new baby and his future and the first: when they know his tragedy in their hearts.

This bridge which links the past with the future can also be applied to the person with CFS. In her or his case we might say that they have two problems: the loss of a healthy life and the acceptance of a difficult and threatening existence. As well as the difficult task of diagnosing CFS, the physician has to help them deal with their loss, help them to accept that life may never be the same for them again and give them hope that they can anticipate a future of increasing ability to cope. The same skills of feeling, thinking, praying and communicating are required and here we will explore the role of the physician as listener and storyteller, In this chapter we will look at the problems and opportunities which arise when the person with CFS goes to see her or his doctor.

To do this it is important to develop the theme of the generalist physician as someone who is there to do much more than use science to diagnose and treat the person with a particular diagnosis or disease. Cassell (1991) has discussed the effect of science on the ideal of the doctor.

> Science attends to objects that are free of value and quality, separate from one another, divorced from the context and times in which they would occur naturally and whose workings can be known by the analysis of their parts.

The results of the research on CFS over the past 10 years are good examples of the problems science can and cannot solve. We now have an agreed classification of the condition and therefore a basis on which research into virology, immunology, endocrinology and psychiatry can be carried out. The results of such research hold out the possibility of producing guidelines as to what management might be successful but the potential benefit is limited because science, in the words of Cassell, cannot deal effectively with individuals, value-laden objects, things that change through time or wholes that are greater than the sum of their parts. The task of the patient–doctor interaction is to use the information gained by science to help the person navigate her or his way through a very chaotic and stormy period of her or his life.

The analogy of the weather is probably a good one, and the generalist and the scientific researcher have a relationship similar to that of the coastguard and the weather forecaster. The latter can forecast patterns but the former has to survive in the midst of potential chaos. Modern generalists have come to believe that science has given them the ability to sit in an office and observe the patient navigate their own way through trouble-free and evidence-based waters. However, the real world still requires hardened veterans who can demonstrate their wisdom, experience, courage and seamanship in extricating people from the shipwrecks of their life and experience. In order to do this successfully, the doctor has to know the rules but also when to ignore them, to improvise and to have a sense of timing and drama. He or she has to balance head, heart and hand (Pellegrino, 1988) by combining knowledge of the science and the patient, compassion for those who are hurting and manual, verbal and dramatic skills.

The doctor 'being there'

> Continuity of care, not unlike the practice of religion, is more than an attendance record. It is the weight of an anchor dropped at the sick bed of a young child, as we attend to her fears and console her mother, and so resist the swift currents of our dutiful day. It is the dogged determination to get to the gist of a patient's story, to be unmistaken about its moral, in order to recognize and rejoin the severed ends of an old man's life. (Loxtercamp, 1991)

Perhaps the most important part of being a doctor in the patient–doctor relationship is being there, which includes all the roles that have to be played such as listener, diagnoser, supporter and manager. Having dropped my anchor at the sick bed of the hundreds of people seen in Dunedin between 1984 and 1992 who had waited an average of 3.7 years before they were given a diagnosis of CFS, it was obvious that something had gone wrong with the patient–doctor relationship. Having listened to the various accounts given by these people, the reasons seemed to be either lack of continuity of care by the same doctor or failure to agree on the cause of the particular symptoms. In the case of Sandy quoted in Chapter 4, the time was only six months but the problem was that she did not agree with the diagnosis of 'exhaustion with anxiety' which her doctor produced. Another patient called Thelma, who waited six years for a diagnosis, said:

> Visits to the doctor brought the reaction that I was suffering from stress. Further visits rewarded me with countless trips to the psychiatrist and three and a half years on antidepressants.

Many hours of discussion with people affected by CFS has indicated that the problem seemed to be that, at least in the context of New Zealand general practice, it was rare for doctors to listen to their patients or to have meaningful dialogue in order to find out what was causing the problem. The difficulty seemed to lie in the one-sidedness of the transaction and in unrealistic expectations on both sides as to the outcome of the investigations. This applied to the testing without truly informed consent, the cursory review of results and the statement that all results are 'normal,' the referral to specialists and the silences of non-diagnosis.

The situation was illustrated at a time when JCM set up group sessions for people with CFS to which other physicians could refer patients. The first of these sessions was a description of the symptoms of CFS. In the group discussion, a 43-year-old teacher said:

> My doctor told me that you were having these sessions and advised me to come along and join. He wouldn't tell me why but now I understand. All you have done is to describe my symptoms – why couldn't he have done that?

The proponents of person-centered care (Stewart *et al.*, 1995) suggest that the exploration of four dimensions of illness experience by physicians will increase patient satisfaction, compliance and recovery time. However, the most important issues are the way doctors perform in the oral tradition and the track record they have over time with the person. People remember their doctors' weaknesses for decades. An octogenarian in Dundee in the 1980s described the attitude of a doctor, long dead, who visited her children in the 1930s:

> He was a very vain man. The first thing he would do when he entered the bedroom was to look for a mirror and check that his hair was in place.

The doctor who has been seeing the person for years has a particular difficulty in these 'bad news' consultations because the person already has fixed views on what kind of person the doctor is. The *abrupt man with no compassion* referred to above was probably like that in every consultation with the mother before the Down's syndrome child was conceived or born. However, even he could have redeemed himself by shedding a tear and saying nothing.

The moment when the doctor provides exactly what the patient needs is the consummate moment in the relationship. Like all forms of art it has to be prepared for, rather than taught or even learned. It is the product of an intact humanity and is not acquired at medical school. Robert Burns (1921) tried to explain these native gifts:

> A set o' dull conceited hashes (useless fellows)
> Confuse their brains in college classes
> They gang (go) in stirks (young cows) and come out asses,
> Plain truth to speak
> An syne (then) they think to climb Parnassus
> By dint o' Greek.

To Burns the poet, the summit of Parnassus was the production of the perfect summing-up in verse of a situation. He compliments the subject, John Lapraik, by saying of his poem:

> I've scarce heard ought described sae weel
> What gen'rous manly bosoms feel

For the family doctor, the summit is the moment of true communication. It is often dependent on several factors being in place, including previous knowledge of the patient, a drama such as childbirth, death or a crash, and an appropriate word or attitude. Patients will often say *I felt she/he really understood what I was going through* and paradoxically will often withhold information from those with whom they don't feel this comfort. A study on the long-term outcome of treatment of headaches (Headache Study Group of the University of Western Ontario, 1986) has shown that the statement by patients that they had been able to discuss their headaches and associated problems fully with the doctor was related to a better outcome. However, few doctors give much credence to this assessment of their attitude as felt by the patient.

Exploring the four dimensions of illness experience will help to make the consultation a truly person-centered experience. The dimensions are:

1 **What do you think is wrong with you?**
   Most people know themselves pretty well and have carefully analyzed their symptoms before they come to see the doctor. It is a pity not to utilize all that wealth of knowledge and experience.

   However, the patient may also come along with a sense of what is 'probably' wrong but wants reassurance that it is not something worse. They want reassurance based on tests or on shared reasoning, not just a patronizing pat on the head. Hence Sandy, the farmer/nurse, wanted to base the decision regarding a possible diagnosis of MS on evidence, not opinion. Any reassurance based on opinion without such evidence had no value.

2 **What are your feelings and fears about this illness?**
   In the first stages of the first crash of an illness like CFS their first feelings are likely to be sheer panic and they might not have a clue as to what is happening. They might also have additional deep fear and anxiety because of the uncontrollable symptoms. Often, people in this situation have themselves 'dead and buried' before they consult with their doctor and it is important to get them to talk openly about their fear of death and disability. Another issue under this heading is to discuss the experience of illness that their family has. For example, a close relative may have had similar symptoms and then went on to have a fatal diagnosis. This kind of disclosure requires an atmosphere of absolute safety and the fact that it does not happen is often diagnostic of the relationship between patient and doctor. So often, the fine porcelain of these feelings and fears in the patient is handed over only to see it dashed on the concrete ideas of the physician.

3 **What effect does the illness have on your functioning?**
   This question is really very important in CFS because the definition requires that significant interference with function is present. If only Dr Rose had asked about Wendy's abilities to cope with the baby and her little boy, about what difficulties there were with Willie, perhaps he would not now be losing her as a patient. The skills in assessing loss of function include the establishment of rapport with the fatigued person and, because such

things as concentration and memory are affected, this will be even more difficult than usual.

4 **What do you expect of me, your doctor?**
The question 'What can I do for you today?' is often the first one asked in a consultation but it is properly the fourth. It will be more fully discussed in the chapter on treatment and will include providing a refuge, advising on validated treatments, symptom control and self-management. The important advantage of the individual and personal doctor is that our role can be a flexible one and that, unlike other sources of help that the person can access, we can offer a unique range of knowledge, skills and care. This advantage can be thrown away if we have the desire to be clever or correct rather than helpful. Also, doctors faced with the multiple needs of the person with CFS will often hear apologies coming from their lips such as 'I'm sorry, all I can do is to offer you support'. It is very important that we have the ability to say that we do not know what to do, and that others may have help when we have none. Honest acknowledgment of ignorance, rather than the authoritative ignorance of pretending to know everything, can often be reassuring and also produces a stimulus to joint exploration for a solution but only if good rapport is established. This approach of *naming* and *framing* is the basis of the reflective approach to practice described by Schon (1986). It is truly medicine at the frontier of knowledge because in it, both doctor and patient are *world-making* and exploring a unique set of circumstances. This is the scary world of acquainting ourselves with the particulars of the patient. We go there armed with a knowledge of the generalities of human disease and human behavior but the knack is to balance these with a large acquaintance with the particulars of the person we meet and the person we are (McWhinney, 1989).

The process of being there is going to take time, and in many cultures, money. However the experience of many patients with CFS is that they waste a lot of time and money in innumerable consultations which seem to be going nowhere, precisely because the story being told is not their story. They are being forced into a pattern that resides in a textbook.

The natural reaction to this state of affairs by patients is to come to the doctor determined to convert him into a proselyte of their own favored theory of illness. However, this would be unnecessary if doctors would listen, take their story and weave it into a joint venture. Listening and then ignoring as irrelevant is worse than not listening at all. Better to have a problem of communication with all its awkwardness because the difficulties indicate it to be a shared process that then can move from being a problem to a healing encounter. The 'difficult patient' will have a reason for hanging on to their version of what it can be, and one of the main ones is that no one has yet been able to offer them a better alternative that explains the symptoms and gives them some way out. In our view, a far more difficult scenario is the 'nice' or 'compliant' patient who agrees with everything the doctor says. The obsession that certain doctors have with the 'heart-sink' patient is an indication of doctor-centeredness and it is interesting that there seems to be no balancing literature on the 'heart-throb' patients, those patients who make the task of the family doctor so worthwhile.

The purpose of this first stage is the melding of the illness experience of the person and the scientific knowledge of the physician into a story. If this story is to remain credible until the moment of healing, according to Brody (1987) it has to have three components.

- It has to be acceptable, given the patient's existing belief system and world view.
- The patient must perceive that he or she is surrounded by and may rely upon a group of caring individuals.
- The patient must achieve a sense of mastery or control over the illness experience either by feeling personally powerful, or by feeling that his or her individual powerlessness can be compensated for by the power of some member of the caring group (such as the physician).

The creation and delivery of an acceptable story requires skills in the oral rather than the written domain and medical students receive very little training in these areas. McWhinney (1984) has written that the bias of our communication is against oral dialogue and in favor of visual display of data and perhaps this is the reason why so many people leave our consultations, determined never to return.

Finding an acceptable explanation

Consultations for Wendy with Dr. Rose must have been such a bore because they never seemed to proceed beyond a struggle to get a diagnosis. Many researchers and observers have decried the desire by people like her to have 'some organic cause' to explain their illness and have claimed that it is a factor in poor prognosis (Aylward, 1996; Joyce et al., 1997). However, we have never met a person who did not believe that their illness was not due to an organic cause. Indeed, the research that seems to have started this myth (Sharpe et al., 1992) was a follow-up of 144 persons who had attended an infectious disease clinic of whom 130 (90%) believed that any infection was the cause. By selecting only the 120 (83%) of these who believed it was a viral infection the writers were able to prove a statistical association with impaired function as measured by a postal questionnaire. Belief in an organic cause is often merely an equal and opposite reaction to the position of 'no cause at all' which seems to be the position of many doctors who, like Dr Rose, are often defended within the narrow confines of their medical universe. He has decided what the diagnosis is according to definitions that are doctor- and disease-centered. Anything outside that frame of reference is 'bizarre, atypical nonsense'. Unable to face the person called Wendy he neutralizes her into 'these people'. Faced with this intransigent stance she has nowhere to go unless he can climb down and meet her on common ground. Although he claims to be 'scientific' his use of pejorative terms such as 'bizarre' and 'atypical' is itself nonsense because he unscientifically wants to claim that all symptoms must be associated with signs that are measurable and observable according to the limited tests he chooses to do. He is not alone in his unscientific position because generations of 'scientists' have followed the absurd position of trying to be objective about subjectivity.

So how do we promote discussion on the nature of the problems that we are trying to solve in the consultation? The simple answer seems to be to ask the patients. In a series of action research studies (Denz-Penhey and Murdoch, 1993; Denz-Penhey et al., 1999) a total of 50 people with CFS in New Zealand spent time negotiating models within which they could explore issues of illness and healing. These would seem to provide a basis on which common ground could be achieved by patients and their doctors.

Their agreed illness model was that CFS was a physical illness with certain symptoms caused by endocrine–immune–system dysfunction or poor capillary blood flow. Further, as it was an illness which had no simple direct treatment, the best hope of getting well was to put the body in the best health condition possible in the hope it would self-heal. The comparison was made with a broken arm. A cast is necessary but the body has to heal itself. Their agreed model of healing was based on a health behavior model in which the person with CFS had to assume responsibility for meeting their own health needs.

Having done that, the group went on to discuss the kinds of services that they really wished from their doctors.

Acknowledgment of the condition

Doctor and patient should agree on a shared paradigm for the problem, otherwise each consultation will end up as a quarrel or a stern lecture with one side not participating. As has been fully outlined in Chapter 1, the international criteria for the symptoms of CFS are now clear and should form the basis of the discussion. As discussed in Chapter 3, there is no proven explanatory model for the problem. However, the doctor's explanation may be that it is *somatized mental disorder* and if he feels strongly, like Dr Rose, that there is no such thing as CFS, then it is unlikely that the relationship can be a healing one. The issues here are clear. The patients don't want this lack of acknowledgment to be a running sore and they want the doctor to have a logical and scientific approach to their continuing care.

An important advance would be studies that enabled doctors and patients to find areas of agreement and disagreement in their view of the illness. A study of the management of Down's syndrome children (Murdoch and Anderson, 1990), comparing the views of their mothers and their physicians, found important differences in perception of what the problems of the families and the role of the physician were. Another complex disorder that has no single cause but seems to represent a personal response to a multitude of biological, psychological, social and cultural factors is depression. A study which compared the views of doctors and patients concerning models for depression (UMDS MSc in General Practice Teaching Group, 1999) found that physicians and patients held similar views about the role of mood-related symptoms, psychological causes and non-medical treatments. However, they varied in that the physicians reported greater support for the importance of somatic symptoms, medical causes and medical treatments. This might explain why patients are reluctant to accept this diagnosis whereas doctors are increasingly aware of the importance of its diagnosis and management to the extent of running national campaigns to defeat depression. The position with CFS seems reversed in that doctors seem reluctant to ascribe importance to somatic features and there are no signs of campaigns by doctors to defeat CFS. The reasons for the differences in acceptability of these two important disorders should be explored, and perhaps discussion might reveal a middle ground which receives the full support of both.

More help with symptom control

Fatigue, headache and muscle pain, depression, anxiety and sleep disturbance are all common symptoms in CFS people. They wanted good advice about how to cope with these and they wanted their doctors to have confidence in their recommendations. They also wanted their feedback about the efficacy or otherwise of any medication to be taken seriously. To be told that the antidepressants were 'working' when they reduced functioning by a further 50% is patently absurd.

They wanted them also to be able to explain the physiological processes involved. As the causes are not known, the physiological process can only be guessed at. However, most doctors can be comfortable in giving an explanation of the hormonal cascade that occurs during the stress response and some general statements as to the inter-relatedness of all body systems. Most participants only wished to be reassured that an explanation was possible, not to be regaled with a detailed account of what actually occurs to produce the symptoms.

A particular issue was that they didn't want their doctors to blame everything on the CFS. They were aware that CFS did not confer immunity to other problems, such as cardiovascular diseases and cancer, and they wanted their doctors to be on the look-out for these.

Advice about improvements in health behaviors

One of the issues here is that most doctors have a very limited range of advice because most are reluctant to advise at all unless they have some 'evidence-based' scientific research to quote from. As has been outlined in Chapter 3, the portfolio of evidence-based research in CFS is small and it is particularly small in the area of the improvement in health behaviors. In contrast, complementary medicine practitioners are not reluctant to discuss these issues and seem unhindered by the lack of research evidence on which to base their claims. Absence of evidence is not evidence of absence and one of the issues not often discussed by proponents of evidence-based medicine is what you do as a doctor if there is no evidence.

The patients know that thus far, there is no simple treatment for this illness. The purpose of these consultations is not scientific research or continuing education. It is not good enough to say 'it's all stress' or 'try these antidepressants'; doctors have to widen their options and explore issues of healing.

General practitioners have been perhaps too eager to refer people with complex disorders like CFS or depression to other professionals, such as psychologists and counselors. This is often done in the false belief that such interventions are helpful in all cases. This optimism may disguise another motive, that such a referral hands these time-consuming problems to someone else. However, there is no evidence that referral to counseling improves outcome in depression (Churchill *et al.*, 1999) and there is also no evidence that depression left undetected does any worse than depression diagnosed and treated (Dowrick and Buchan, 1995; Goldberg *et al.*, 1998). What is obvious is that all these complex disorders result in a chronic illness with considerable physical and psychological disabilities in more than 50% of people if they and their doctors do not attempt to correct the underlying issues.

The groups felt that they should not be forced into a decision between mind and body as the source and explanation for their illness. Their view was that this was often insisted on by doctors. They were aware of the importance of anger, grief and stress management, the need to improve ways of coping, working at relationships and developing improved communication skills but didn't see that they had to 'confess' to having psychological problems in order to access these. They also knew that any psychological diagnoses are carried for life and have to be 'confessed' on insurance and job application forms forever, with detrimental effects financially and workwise. They were extremely untrusting of the psychological establishment and it is interesting that in the questionnaire study, the psychiatrist was regarded as the most unhelpful of all the professionals consulted.

The measurement of psychopathology contains more than a hint of confession with the associated guilt and blame but without the absolution. The General Health Questionnaire may be interpreted by doctors as a valid instrument to measure depression but the need to have a uniform scoring system seems to deny any concept of finding common ground, and gives all the power to the scorer.

Relapse prevention

This was recognized as important by the group but was not discussed in great detail.

The ultimate responsibility in family medicine is to the patient and the outcome which we have to seek in practice is 'the best we can do in the circumstances'. The ground of our being is on the level of the patient, in the swampy ground of reality and not up on the high ground of what Schon (1986) calls 'technical rationality.' We all know that in 'an ideal world' we would prefer to make a definite diagnosis and apply an evidence-based treatment if any is proven by randomized controlled trials. In most of these situations, even the diagnosis is uncertain and the progress will only come by reflection on the circumstances and by the improvisations of artists on both sides of the relationship. Schon (1986) likens the medical practitioner to a musical performer.

> Musical performance is a kind of designing. It is true that the performer has access to a score which gives him the pitches and durations to be played, along with the indications of fingerings, *legato* and *staccato* playing, dynamics, tempo, and such expressive descriptions as *furioso* or *andante cantabile*. But the performer also has a great deal of discretion.

The challenge of the interaction between the doctor and the person with CFS is of a strange and difficult score with considerable demands on interpretation and performance. The story told by countless thousands of CFS patients is of practitioners who seem afraid to leave their theories behind and reach out to embrace the person and escort her or him to better health. In fact, the stories are of supposed performers who cannot play at all.

Surrounded by care: matching the whole persons of the doctor and the patient

In our case study, Dr Alan Rose, as a person, has some problems with Wendy Jones as a newly ill person. Before, it didn't seem to matter but now it does. Traditionally doctors have regarded themselves as neutral or objective in the relationship but manifestly this cannot be so. Dr Rose is male, middle-aged, apparently healthy, seemingly married to a healthy woman who has had one child who has been healthy too, as far as we know. Wendy is female, young, sick, married to a potentially alcoholic husband and has two young children whom she is unable to look after. Dealing with him as a person, for Wendy, is like dealing with her own father. This is a problem, but not an insuperable one, provided that Dr Rose understands the position he is in.

Many doctors like Dr Rose have an over-inflated view of their reputations with their patients. Most of us would cringe if we knew what our patients said about us to their nearest and dearest after they returned home from the consultation. When one of the authors (JCM) was leaving his first practice after eight years, an 85-year-old lady whom he had visited monthly for that time had this to say about his contribution to her life:

> What a pity that you are leaving, doctor, just as everybody was beginning to like you.

When doctors go into practice, they often inherit the myths and legends which have accompanied the healer over the centuries. Many people still talk about 'the doctor' and put the person who is the doctor on a professional pedestal. Whatever reasons they may have for doing this, difficulties arise when the doctor begins to believe in these myths and legends. Like the newly crowned Emperors of Rome, they need to be reminded that they, too, are persons, and vulnerable persons, given their high rates of psychiatric illness and addictive behaviors.

Underneath that gruff exterior, Alan Rose's biography would surprise his patients. He was an only son whose father died when he was 16, and his mother worked her fingers to the bone to save the money to send him to university. Fortunately, in those days there was a socialist government and he got a scholarship to support him for the six years of his course. His wife, Cynthia, was an arts student three years younger than him whom he met at a student dance. They became very close and unfortunately she became pregnant as these were the days before the contraceptive pill and abortion. Of course, it caused a real fuss in both families, particularly Cynthia's. Her father was a successful industrialist and her mother a socialite. Since they were both so very young, they were persuaded to have the baby adopted, so that they could finish their degrees and get married at their leisure. They were married two years after he qualified and once he had completed four years as a registrar, his father-in-law gave him the money to buy his family practice. They then settled down to have a family but their first child was stillborn. Cynthia then had two miscarriages and their only daughter was born after a traumatic pregnancy during which Cynthia vomited continuously and the child was born by cesarian section. Since then Cynthia Rose has suffered from chronic anxiety and has been in and out of psychiatric hospitals. Alan has struggled along to bring up his daughter and support his wife. His daughter has now left home, and when last heard of was bumming her way round the States with a rock musician who was very much part of the drug scene. Not surprisingly, Mrs Rose has been even more upset and Dr Rose's nurse has to field many calls in the day so that his consulting is not interrupted. His mother, Mrs Rose Senior, is in an old people's home but he never has the time to visit her.

All this is apocryphal but it could be true. Dr Rose would never breathe a word of it to any of his patients and yet he would expect to ask all these questions of people who present to him with long-standing symptoms like Wendy. He, too, is a parent, a partner, a son and he has a past, a present and a future. All these facts about him are relevant to his management of his patients but he has learned to hide them all in his dealings with them. He found when he first dealt with people in medical school that he was too sensitive to the pain and feelings of others and he had learnt over time to hide his 'problem' by adopting the professional manner he saw in senior doctors at his teaching hospital. Many of his patients worship his professional manner, his impeccable dress, his faultless manners. Don't get us wrong, it's not that Wendy would rather he dropped the front and revealed his shyness, his embarrassment, his family difficulties. She probably does not mind all that front and wants her doctor to be all-knowing and kindly. What she also wants is that he develop awareness and that he should not project his wife's problems on to her. He does not believe that his wife makes enough effort, she's too dependent, whereas Wendy's problem is that she tries too hard, does not spend enough time looking after herself and is too independent. She wants to manage without help and does not seek help at an early stage.

Dr John Sassall, the subject of a famous book on general practice, mused thoughtfully about this issue.

> Sassall is acknowledged as a good doctor because he meets the deep but unformulated expectation of the sick for a sense of fraternity. He recognizes them. Sometimes he fails, often because he has missed a critical opportunity and the patient's suppressed resentment becomes too hard to break through, but there is about him the constant will of a man trying to recognize. 'The door opens', he says, 'and sometimes I feel as if I'm in the valley of death. It's all right when once I'm working. I try to overcome this shyness because

> for the patient the first contact is extremely important. If he's put off and doesn't feel welcome, it may take a long time to win his confidence back and perhaps never. I try to give him a fully open greeting. All diffidence in my position is a fault. A form of negligence'. (Berger, 1967)

Diffidence isn't the only problem, of course. Arrogance and the need to control in such a way that requires patient submission and obedience is the opposite end of the spectrum. According to Sassall, the battle for the confidence of Wendy by Dr Rose was lost many years before, when he discovered diffidence as the cure for his shyness. Dr Rose does not realize that his diffidence may be a polite form of arrogance. That is the problem. This negligence is revealed when he greeted her for the first time in this illness with a quiet 'What can I do for you today?' instead of 'Wendy, come in, how are the children, you look very tired, what's the problem?' Or was it when he coldly told her, 'All the tests are normal, there's nothing wrong with you', when she was sitting there with pale face drawn with pain and fatigue and unable to think clearly about how she was going to manage the drive home, let alone how she could manage shopping for food for tea on the way.

Sassall, too, was an old fashioned doctor, a bit like Dr Rose, but for him the person-centered approach was the antidote to his shyness.

> Sassall needs to work in this way. He cures others to cure himself. (Berger, 1967)

There are three things that can be changed as a doctor meets a patient in a consultation. The first is the illness which can be diagnosed, treated and prognosed, and the second and third are the personalities of the patient and the doctor which can be transformed through the relationship. Doctors often forget that we can be changed too.

Janet Frame, one of New Zealand's most distinguished writers spent seven years of her 20s in psychiatric hospitals in New Zealand where she was diagnosed as suffering from chronic schizophrenia. During that time she met many doctors and was able to use her memories of the locked ward to describe some of them in her novels.

> The chief of the white tribe, who wore spectacles, and carried in his pocket the sprout of a rubber tree to listen at the underground door of the heart and its beating of secret, walked forward and smiled encouragingly, saying – Now now, Daphne, speak to me like a good girl. We are going to make you better after all this time. You'll be home soon.

What was intended was a frontal leucotomy and later in the book, the doctor returns to tell her what is going to happen.

> Well, Daphne, the doctor said. You're going to have some visitors. Your brother and father. You'll like that, won't you? And tomorrow we're going to take you for a ride in a car, to another hospital, and you're going to go to sleep, and wake up better. We're going to change you so that you'll be able to live in the world and be just like other people, and you'll like that, won't you? (Frame, 1961)

In real life, Janet and literature were spared the ordeal of the leucotomy but not 200 applications of electroconvulsive therapy. A few years later, having established herself as a writer of merit, she came to Europe and was seen as an inpatient in the Maudsley Hospital by Dr. Robert Cawley, at that time a psychiatric registrar. He describes his attempt to examine her mental state.

> Nature, said Bacon, is more infinite in her manifestations than man in his conceptions. It is hardly surprising that the formalised attempt to comprehend a person's mental state ... may sometimes seem, if not completely futile, rather laughable. Perhaps this was the first thing I learned from Janet Frame. There I sat with this quiet, nervous, enigmatic woman, writing my observations as I plied her with the standard questions. It soon emerged that an instrument of clinical investigation was meeting some powerful resistance from a force which could perhaps challenge and debunk much of what I believed I knew. And as I proceeded, the patient became rather dogged, more alert, more confident. Her eyes brightened. She was responding more than I had thought she might, but in a different way. I perceived that there were things to be learned and un-learned from this friendly mystery person who appeared to be conducting a teaching session: it was as if she hoped to illuminate the matter in hand by recourse to a kind of mocking scepticism. (Cawley, 1994)

Janet's view of the same interview was rather different. In her autobiography she talked of her pleasure that the psychiatrist had trained in zoology and mathematics before doing medicine, unlike her previous psychiatrist, Dr Portion.

> The qualifications of medicine and psychiatry were extensions of these men, not starting and ending points. I had felt that although Dr Portion was a qualified psychiatrist, he may have superimposed life upon psychiatry and not psychiatry upon life.

However, her first impressions of Dr Cawley were not good.

> I was disconcerted when during our first interview Dr Cawley sat with pen and paper and wrote or appeared to write everything I said without looking up ... I guessed he might have been a shy man ... He spoke with an 'English'

accent that chilled me whenever I heard it in the distance but in his presence it could not frighten me for he was not aggressive, his manner was excessively polite, his smile kindly as if these were more a protection for himself than a gift for me. I felt he was a clever, uncertain man whose sole triumph in our interviews was the accuracy of his recording the content.

However, over time the relationship grew and the healing occurred.

> With time, the marvellous luxury of time, and patience, Dr Cawley convinced me that I was myself, an adult, I need not explain myself to others ... I now had confidence in Dr Cawley, for I had not only seen myself developing and growing in his care, I had observed his own development as an assured psychiatrist who, I felt, would always respect the human spirit before the practice, the fashions and the demands of psychiatry. I was influenced also by the persistence of Dr Cawley in being 'himself' and not some 'image' of a psychiatrist: he did not patronise or pretend, and when he talked of my writing, he confessed modestly, with the old-fashioned air of someone from a Somerset Maugham story, 'I'm not a literary chap, you know.' No longer, I hoped, dependent on my 'schizophrenia' for comfort and attention and help, but with myself as myself, I again began my writing career. (Frame, 1985)

People with CFS bring a person as well as a diagnosis to the consultation and part of our task is to find that person and to unearth the positive aspects so that the relationship can be fruitful. The term 'heartsink' for the difficult patient betrays the fact that the real problem for many doctors is that they cannot find much of a person to admire in the patient. In fact, the person with CFS often shares the doctor's view that they are useless and unattractive. Work often needs to be done to encourage a positive and adaptive coping mechanism and to underline the fact that an attractive personality is possible in spite of symptoms. However, the important points which emerge from the interaction between Frame and Cawley is that it is just as healing for the doctor as it is for the patient. This surrounding with care, the meeting of two souls, far from being an exhausting process is a reviving and a developing process for the doctor.

Helping the person to achieve a sense of mastery and control

The most important result of the meeting between Dr Cawley and Janet Frame was the fact that she was able to take charge of her life and resume her writing career. She was able to do that through a process which required great patience on both sides. As we have seen there is still much controversy about the natural history of CFS with some studies showing that the majority of people eventually improve and others showing that only a minority do. We can only guess at what the mechanism of recovery is, but what is clear is that it results from changes in physical and emotional functioning.

One of the problems which we have as doctors is that we have been trained in diagnosis rather than applying ourselves to therapeutic situations. Accordingly, we become easily bored with situations where there is a lack of action or progress. It took time and patience to allow Janet Frame to achieve mastery of her life and we need to examine ways of assisting the process of healing through the patient–physician relationship.

Conclusion: enjoying the physician–patient relationship in chronic fatigue syndrome

Part of the problem which doctors and patients have in the meetings which they have with each other is that neither particularly enjoys the experience. Those with CFS are 'difficult patients'.

> The despair, anger, and frustration that we feel with certain patients is part of our everyday lives; we are all familiar with that feeling which overwhelms us when we see Mr or Ms X's name in the visit book. (Gerrard and Riddell, 1988)

Most of the writings in the medical literature see these issues from the doctor's point of view. We hear little of the despair, anger and frustration felt by Mr or Ms X as they sit in the doctor's waiting room. These problems often arise in doctors from unresolved emotions such as guilt at not being able to understand what is going on in this patient and inability to help relieve the symptoms. From the patients point of view there is also guilt at 'wasting the doctor's time' with a problem he or she does not understand and frustration at the time it is taking to improve. If these emotional issues are not shared, something sooner or later has got to give, as it did between Wendy and Dr Rose, and it is important that both doctors and patients are able to communicate their true feelings on the subject.

If only Dr Rose had been able to say out loud what he was thinking and feeling about Wendy's situation, perhaps the situation might have been different.

One of the problems lies in what Patch Adams (Adams and Mylander 1993) has called *the distance ethic*; maintaining a scientist's detachment and dealing with patients as if they were experiments in a laboratory.

The relationship deepens if the patient knows as much about me, the physician, as I know about him or her. If the relationship is steeped in friendship, love, mutuality, caring and fun, then the time spent together can evolve into a partnership where each is vulnerable to and trusts the other. This intimacy is the bedrock of burnout-free practice.

Most of medicine today is run as a business and we need to realize as medical practitioners and as business people that the distance which we insert between ourselves and our patients constitutes a bar to successful operating. Like many other businesses our medical practices have a learning disability and they need to become what Senge (1990) has called 'learning organizations'. What Senge has described as the cardinal features of unprofitable companies are all there to be seen. As doctors, we play an authoritative role which is outmoded in the modern world. We have the illusion of being in charge and we have not noticed that most of the people who need our help are going elsewhere. Many of our problems would be solved if we could dismantle the one-way screen which lies between our side of the desk and our patient. People don't want the distance ethic, they want honest, human and realistic people to help them through their difficulties.

References

Adams P and Mylander M (1993) *Gesundheit! Bringing Good Health to You, the Medical System and Society through Physician Service, Complementary Therapies, Humor and Joy.* Healing Arts Press, Rochester, VT.

Aylward M (1996) Government's expert group has reached consensus on prognosis of chronic fatigue syndrome. *BMJ.* **313**: 885.

Berger J (1967) *A Fortunate Man: the story of a country doctor.* The Penguin Press, London, UK.

Brody H (1987) *Storytelling in Medicine in Stories of Sickness.* Yale University Press, New Haven, CT.

Burns R (1921) Epistle to John Lapraik, an old Scottish Bard. In: JL Robertson (ed.) *The Poetical Works of Robert Burns.* Oxford University Press, London, UK.

Cassell EJ (1991) *The Nature of Suffering and the Goals of Medicine.* Oxford University Press, Oxford, UK.

Cox H (1973) *Seduction of the Spirit: the use and misuse of people's religion.* Simon & Schuster, New York.

Cawley R (1994) Janet Frame's contribution to the education of a psychiatrist. In: E Alley (ed.) *The Inward Sun: celebrating the life and work of Janet Frame.* Daphne Brasell Associates Press. Wellington, NZ.

Churchill R, Dewey M, Gretton V et al. (1999) Should general practitioners refer patients with major depression to counsellors?: a review of current published evidence. *Br J Gen Pract*. 49: 737–43.

Denz-Penhey H and Murdoch JC (1993) Service delivery for people with chronic fatigue syndrome: a pilot action research study. *Fam Pract*. 10: 14–18.

Denz-Penhey H, Tilyard MW, Shaw R and Harvey R (1999) Patient self-management in chronic fatigue syndrome: an action research study. *NZ Fam Physician*. 26: 43–50.

Dowrick C and Buchan I (1995) Twelve-month outcome of depression in general practice: does detection or disclosure make a difference? *BMJ*. 311: 1274–6.

Franklin AW (1958) Care of the mongol baby. *Lancet*. 1: 256–8.

Frame J (1961) *Owls Do Cry*. Random Century New Zealand Ltd, Auckland, NZ.

Frame J (1985) *The Envoy from Mirror City*. Random Century New Zealand Ltd, Auckland, NZ.

Gerrard TJ and Riddell JD (1988) Difficult patients: black holes and secrets. *BMJ*. 297: 530–2.

Goldberg D, Privett M, Ustun B, Simon G and Linden M (1998) The effects of the detection and treatment on the outcome of major depression in primary care: a naturalistic study in 15 cities. *Br J Gen Pract*. 48: 1840–4.

Headache Study Group of the University of Western Ontario (1986) Predictors of outcome in headache patients presenting to family physicians: a one year prospective study. *Headache*. 26: 285–94.

Joyce J, Hotopf M and Wessely S (1997) The prognosis of chronic fatigue and chronic fatigue syndrome: a systematic review. *Q J Med*. 90: 223–33.

Loxtercamp D (1991) Being there: on the place of the family physician. *J Am Board Fam Pract*. 4: 354–60.

McWhinney IR (1984) Changing models: the impact of Kuhn's theory on medicine. *Fam Pract*. 1: 3–8.

McWhinney IR (1989) 'An acquaintance with particulars...' *Fam Med*. 21: 296–8.

Marinker M (1983) Communication in general practice. In: D Pendleton and J Hasler (eds) *Doctor–Patient Communication*. Academic Press, London, UK.

Murdoch JC (1984) Experience of the mothers of Down's syndrome and spina bifida children on going home from hospital in Scotland 1971–81. *J Ment Def Res*. 28: 123–7.

Murdoch JC and Anderson VE (1990) The management of Down's syndrome children and their families in general practice. In: WI Fraser (ed.) *Key Issues in Mental Retardation Research*. Routledge, London and New York.

Pellegrino ED (1988) Balancing head, heart and hand in the physician's education: a special task for family practice. *J Am Board Fam Pract*. 1: 4–14.

Schon DA (1986) *Educating the Reflective Practitioner*. Jossey-Bass Publishers, San Francisco, CA.

Senge PM (1990) *The Fifth Discipline: the art and practice of the learning organization.* Doubleday, New York.

Sharpe M, Hawton K, Seagrott, V and Pasvol G (1992) Follow-up of patients presenting with fatigue to an infectious diseases clinic. *BMJ.* **305**: 147–52.

Stewart M, Brown JB, Weston WW *et al.* (1995) *Patient-Centered Medicine: transforming the clinical method.* Sage Publications, Thousand Oaks, CA.

UMDS MSc General Practice Teaching Group (1999) 'You're depressed': 'No, I'm not': GPs' and patients' different models of depression. *Br J Gen Pract.* **49**: 123–4.

Finding the appropriate treatment for chronic fatigue syndrome

Case study
Wendy's new physician, Dr Monica Lane, listened while Wendy told her at length about how her illness had affected her and described her most difficult symptoms. She reviewed her investigations and suggested there was enough evidence there to rule out any other cause for her symptoms. She agreed that it sounded as though the most likely diagnosis was CFS. She asked Wendy what she thought would be the best way to proceed and they agreed that they should give priority to symptom control and managing the effects of the crash. She explained to Wendy why she felt so ill. She recommended that she had help at home and put her in touch with the local CFS support group.

Dr Lane and Wendy agreed that she would have a consultation every two weeks to discuss symptom control and deal with any problems that arose. She was comfortable that Wendy consult a naturopath to discuss nutritional modifications and avoidance of foods that seemed to make certain symptoms worse. She also offered to meet with Willie and answer any questions that he might have. A year later, Wendy is feeling much better although she has some bad days with her old symptoms and feels reluctant to declare herself cured.

People with the terrible symptoms that make up the diagnosis of CFS usually have only two questions which they wish to ask about the disorder. The first is 'What caused it?' and the second is 'How do I get rid of it?' Unlike the health professionals who are interested in the problem, their interest is not academic or intellectual but personal and many of them are so desperate that they would try literally anything and go anywhere to find some respite from their problems. It is very difficult to convey the compelling nature of these symptoms. As one sufferer in Dunedin wrote in 1983:

It is difficult to adequately explain the general feeling of ME. It is the most distressing symptom of all but seems to be common to all sufferers. A possible way to duplicate this feeling might be:

- wait till you catch flu
- drink copious quantities of cheap whisky and wine
- work hard physically all day
- stay up all night
- go to bed and set the alarm for three hours sleep.

When you awake you will have something approaching the ME feeling.

Through the course of this book we have outlined the case for this disorder being distinct from others and it is now clear that no person should ever be told that there is no such condition as CFS. The days of waiting many years for a diagnosis should hopefully now be over. However, while there is evidence that doctors are now more willing to accept the concept, patients often meet another hurdle, which is to be told that there is no treatment for CFS. What the people who say this mean is that there is no drug which has been proven to 'switch off' the symptoms of CFS, and the statement is only true in that context.

So again we come to a philosophical problem which has existed in the medical profession and indeed in the whole human race for thousands of years. From time immemorial there has been a conflict between those doctors who understand illness as a result of the convergence of disease, personal and environmental factors in an individual, and those who believe that illness is caused by factors outside of individual or environmental control. The latter kind of doctor looks for faulty parts in the body machine and either removes or replaces them or gets round the malfunction by giving the patient drugs of some kind. It is this kind of doctor who most usually says that there is no treatment for CFS. The former kind of doctor will regard cause as important in some illnesses but will also know that attention to the personal and environmental issues will also improve the chances of healing in the life of the affected individual.

The practice of patient-centered medicine is a commitment to people and not to diseases. We have spent a lot of time in this book demonstrating that CFS can be categorized and there has been a lot of research effort put into trying to demonstrate a cause, but in some ways that should not matter. The patient-centered doctor should be able to treat those people who come to him or her, irrespective of age, sex or category of illness. Uncertainty about diagnosis should be a joy to us, not a difficulty.

Under the heading of 'treatment' there should be agreement on which tasks are better done by the doctors, which by the patient and what, if anything, might be better handled by those who practice complementary therapies. Chronic illness and its management belongs to the patient and not to the doctor and the successful patient–doctor relationship will result in the patient making the decisions and the choices. This chapter will, therefore, primarily be concerned with the following issues: the importance of providing a refuge for the patient, naming the problem of CFS, a short summary of the scientifically validated treatments, patient self-management, continuing care, shared care and what to do when there is no improvement.

Refuge provision

We use the term 'refuge' as meaning a place of shelter from pursuit, danger or trouble. In our experience, most people with CFS approach their doctor in great distress at the puzzling and disabling symptoms that have overtaken them. The symptoms of the disorder often make them confused with loss of concentration and short-term memory. Like all people who are ill they feel isolated and this is often made worse by the difficulty doctors have in naming their illness. Berger (1967) commented that illness separates and encourages a distorted, fragmented form of self-consciousness.

The first work to be done is to offer a refuge, a place of safety, where the account of their symptoms can be heard, believed and accepted and where there can be rest from the incessant insistence on quick fixes and cures. This is a sensitive and fragile occasion, akin to the first interview with a rape victim. It is a time for positive, unconditional regard. To Berger (1967) again:

> The doctor, through his relationship with the invalid and by means of the special intimacy he is allowed, has to compensate for these broken connections and reaffirm the social content of the invalid's aggravated self-consciousness.

Those who have cared for many hundreds of CFS patients have experienced the sense of relief felt by these people when they realize that this particular consultation is not a medical quiz game with the winner announced after blood tests, but an affirmation of a recognizable and believable set of circumstances. Stott (1983) has classified the role of the refuge in clinical practice as:

1 a primary refuge from distressing symptoms and from fear of serious disease, providing reassurance, symptom relief and cures
2 a secondary refuge when official sanction of the sick role is required by society to provide proof of *bona fide* illness which prevents patients from fulfilling their social functions
3 a tertiary refuge when the distressed and/or diseased person needs hospital care, a hospice or a place of safety for healing, relief or protection.

Physicians and other professionals running services for CFS will need to provide a primary and a secondary refuge. Tertiary refuges are few and far between but have an important role in the management of those with severe CFS. There should be an unwritten rule that these doctors and their staff should treat those patients who consult them with positive and unconditional regard. Professionals who are rude and insulting to those who have undiagnosed symptoms, and regard them as figures of fun should have no place in their treatment. Of course it is said that 'there is a danger that if such a refuge for people with CFS is provided, this will make them dependent'. This theory is also used in much the same way with regard to providing narcotic drugs to those who are in extreme pain. There may come a time when dependency will be a problem, perhaps a time for straight talking, just as there might be in any condition such as cancer or rheumatoid arthritis, but this is not the time.

It is fascinating to discuss why this most obvious step, of providing a refuge to those who are so obviously sick, is often omitted in the case of CFS. Part of the problem lies in our lack of understanding of people in this position and a selective approach to those whom we think deserve compassionate care. Most doctors are compassionate to the dying and the obviously diseased but this is often because of pity for their poor prognosis and recognizable pain. Fox (1979) points out that such pity works out of a subject–object relationship where what is primary is one's separateness from another. People do not need pity, but compassion. Doctors have no training in how to understand and live compassion as a way of practice. The closest we can get to even a memory of it is in the religious life and the works of mercy which were feeding, clothing, sheltering, setting- free, giving drink, visiting, burying, educating, counseling, admonishing, bearing wrongs, forgiving, comforting and praying. As other secular institutions, medicine has proved itself incapable of performing these works of mercy and compassion and in that failure lies much of the pain in our world. Perhaps we need the spirit of a Mother Teresa (Egan, 1985) whose accolade was that she advanced peace by her extraordinary reaffirmation of the inviolability of human dignity. Compassion, as Fox (1979) points out, is justice-making and at the root of this problem with CFS and other undiagnosable diseases is prejudice. Nothing else could explain the terms such as 'dependent clingers', 'entitled demanders', 'manipulative help-rejectors' and 'self-destructive deniers' used by doctors to describe people who challenge their abilities by failing to recover. The use of these terms indicates that the patients have become objects, not subjects and those who use the terms are affected by a tendency to ego-defense and invulnerability.

Agreeing a name for the problem

It is obvious that much of the reason for the lack of confidence between patients and doctors is the lack of agreement about the diagnosis and the consequent conflict surrounding the right for the patient to be ill. As a result of this disagreement the relationship will always be in crisis. For the doctor it may be an intellectual issue but for the patient it is a personal one and the doctor's refusal to give a diagnosis will be interpreted as a refusal to acknowledge that the patient is ill. Even where the doctor cannot believe that the symptoms relate to a definite disease, progress could be made if he or she could at least agree that there is a problem and both parties could then agree what to call it.

The initial consultation should be long (at least 30 minutes). It should include a full history and physical examination, and since the patient will often have spent a long time wandering in the wilderness of non-diagnosis, should be focussed on ending with at least a provisional opinion on diagnosis, i.e. the clear opinion of the reviewer as to whether the assessment indicates whether the person has CFS according to the international criteria. A written statement of the international criteria as contained in Chapter 1 might also be shared and given to the patient as a confirmation. As we have already said, it should not be too difficult to classify the story into CFS, IFS or to suggest that some other diagnosis exists.

What are the scientifically validated treatments?

Doctors, so the story goes, are supposed to make you better, and the next stage of treatment for the orthodox physician would normally be to apply a treatment that had been evaluated in clinical trial. However, as we have already seen in Chapter 3 the physiological mechanisms which cause the symptoms of CFS are still a matter of dispute. Some doctors believe that the problem is triggered by a virus leading to an abnormal immune response, others that the symptoms are caused by depression and other psychological factors, others that the problem is due to abnormalities in hypothalamo–pituitary–adrenal function and a few who believe that the symptoms are due to poor capillary blood flow.

One of the roles of scientific academic research is to devise treatments that are thought to modify these mechanisms and to test them out by randomizing a number of patients to the treatment or placebo (an inert substance given in place of the real thing) and then measuring whether there is a difference in the symptoms. The same process can also be done by doing what are called 'N of 1' studies where the treatment and placebo are rotated in the same patient (Guyatt et al., 1986). The randomized controlled trials (RCTs) are the 'gold standard' of absolute proof that the treatment works. Normally, governments will only fund treatments that pass this very rigorous test and also the test that the drug will not do harm due to its chemical characteristics.

The RCTs that have been done in CFS have looked at many varied treatments which have largely reflected the theories of causation which were described in Chapter 3. The results to date have been summarized in a recent review (Reid et al., 2000). This has reported on the research to date on certain interventions that have been studied and found to be helpful.

Graded exercise programs

There have been two RCTs of graded exercise programs in CFS (Fulcher and White, 1997; Weardon et al., 1998) the first involving 66 people and the second 136. Some may quibble over whether these are really RCTs because the 'placebo' in the first was flexibility training and in the second was no exercise at all. The paper describing this second study makes the hilarious comment that 'patients were blind to assignment to exercise or appointments'.

Both studies found that the people assigned to exercise programs had substantially improved measures of fatigue and physical functioning. However, 37% of the people assigned to exercise in the second trial withdrew as opposed to 22% of those in the appointments group.

Exercise programs were first introduced for the treatment of tuberculosis in 19th century sanatoria and recent research has shown it to be helpful in varied disorders, such as cardiac and respiratory disease. The reviewers warn against overambitious and overhasty attempts at exercise and it should be remembered that these trials were well-planned and professionally supervised. Anecdotal evidence suggests that many people with CFS are tempted to over-exercise with a view to proving that they are not really ill or that they really are trying and not 'playing ill'.

Cognitive behavioral therapy

The greatest number of RCTs have been carried out into this intervention which is a form of psychotherapy. Three trials were included, two of which showed benefit (Deale et al., 1997; Lloyd et al., 1993; Sharpe et al., 1996.) However, the trials which showed the most benefit (Deale et al., 1997; Sharpe et al., 1996) were those in which the intervention was delivered by what are termed 'highly skilled behavioural therapists' and the programs were intensive with 16 one-hour individual treatment sessions over four months.

Antidepressants

There have been two RCTs of the use of fluoxetine (Vercoulen et al., 1996; Weardon et al., 1998) in CFS. The first of these found no benefit even when the patients were depressed. The second showed a beneficial effect only at 12 weeks in the 26-week trial. There was also an RCT of low-dose phenelzine, a monoamine oxidase inhibitor, in CFS which produced a non-significant pattern of improvement over only six weeks (Natelson et al., 1996).

Corticosteroids

Limited data from three trials on fludrocortisone, (Peterson et al., 1998) hydrocortisone 25–35 mg daily (McKenzie et al., 1998) and hydrocortisone 5–10 mg (Cleare et al., 1999) showed that any benefit was short-lived and that higher doses were associated with adverse effects, such as adrenal depression.

Dietary supplements such as magnesium and efamol

Results of the trials of Efamol have been found to be conflicting, with one claiming benefit (Behan et al., 1990) and the other not (Warren et al., 1999). A study which found levels of magnesium to be low in CFS patients has not been able to be replicated (Cox et al., 1991).

Energy-providing substances

A trial of oral nicotinamide adenine dinucleotide (NADH) which facilitates the generation of ATP, a major source of energy within cells, showed benefit over placebo (Forsyth et al., 1999).

Another substance responsible for mitochondrial energy production is L-carnitine. For some reason, this was compared with amantadine which has been effective in treating the fatigue seen in multiple sclerosis patients. L-carnitine was found to be more effective than amantadine in CFS patients but amantadine was poorly tolerated and only half the patients were able to tolerate the treatment (Plioplys and Plioplys, 1997).

Antiviral and immunoregulatory drugs

The use of these treatments stemmed from the theory that CFS symptoms were due to defects of immune regulation. In spite of initial optimism the use of intravenous infusions of immunoglobulin has now been proved to be ineffective, at least in adults (Lloyd et al., 1990; Peterson at al., 1990; Vollmer-Conna et al., 1997). A trial in adolescents showed benefit over placebo solution but both the treated groups and the placebo groups made excellent progress (Rowe, 1997). One trial (See and Tilles, 1996) found benefit from interferon alfa but only in those patients with an isolated decrease in natural killer cell function. In another trial (Strayer et al., 1994) a specifically configured RNA drug with antiviral and immunomodulatory properties (Ampligen) was shown to improve energy, exercise capacity, reduce cognitive deficit and improve the activities of daily living more than placebo. Another antiviral drug called acyclovir was shown to have no benefit in improving the symptoms of CFS (Straus et al., 1988).

Vitamin B12

The use of injections of vitamin B12 for those who suffer from fatigue has been going on for many years. It has been estimated to be used by general practitioners up to 20 times more than would be justified for the treatment of pernicious anemia (Cochrane and Moore, 1971). A placebo-controlled cross-over study of B12 injections in people with chronic tiredness (Ellis and Nasser, 1973) was made more difficult by the possible persistence of the effect of the active component into the placebo phase. However, those who were on placebo first showed beneficial effects from the B12 injections. The interest in B12 in CFS comes from its use in the treatment of neuropsychiatric disorders in the absence of anemia or macrocytosis (Lindebaum et al., 1988), and in the finding that vitamin B12 deficiency has been found associated with neurological dysfunction in human immunodeficiency virus infection (Kieburtz et al., 1991). Although B12 injections have been used widely in CFS patients, there has been no formal trial. Anecdotal evidence suggests that about a third of people seem to be improved. The only trial in CFS was of a liver extract–folic acid–cyanocobalamin extract which showed no benefit over placebo after four weeks (Kaslow et al., 1989).

Conclusions from the scientific research

It is obviously important to do research studies so that we can demonstrate which interventions are proven in the management of people with CFS. However, in order to do a RCT, we have to understand the processes which are being treated and that is obviously not possible with CFS because no one yet understands why people become ill in this way. The trials so far conducted have only involved a total of 1000–2000 people and they have been selected because they attended the specialized clinics of those who were doing the research. Even when the CDC criteria are applied and it is known that the people selected have CFS, the outcome measurements are increases or decreases in symptom scores and on self-rated questionnaires. These are usually summated into global scores and it seems rather naive to equate statistical improvements in global scores with efficacy of the drug or management under scrutiny. This impression is underlined by the fact that RCTs in CFS have tended to produce conflicting results.

The superficial assessment of these studies conducted so far would suggest that cognitive behavioral therapy and graduated exercise programs are the most successful ways of treating people with CFS but a deeper look at both these modalities underlines the difficulty of generalizing the results of these studies to the worldwide population of CFS sufferers.

Cognitive behavioral therapy (CBT) is a form of psychotherapy which has been used primarily for psychological disorders and its use has been developed and studied by those who believe that CFS is a psychiatric disorder. In the introduction to their RCT on cognitive behavioral therapy Sharpe and his colleagues (1996) tell us that:

> Cognitive behavioral therapy offers a novel approach to treatment of the chronic fatigue syndrome. It is based on the hypothesis that inaccurate and unhelpful beliefs, ineffective coping behavior, negative mood states, social problems, and pathophysiological processes all interact to perpetuate the illness. Treatment aims at helping patients to re-evaluate their understanding of the illness and to adopt more effective coping behaviors.

This seems to us to offer a very negative view of the person with CFS and one wonders whether informed consent was received with respect to this hypothesis before the trial commenced. Furthermore, one of the desired outcomes of the study was to effect a change in beliefs about the illness. For example, at the outset 83% of the 30 people given CBT believed that their illness was mainly physical and 63% called it ME. After 16 one-hour individual treatment sessions with one of three skilled behavioral therapists, only 33% still thought it was mainly a physical illness and 17% called it ME. On the other hand, whereas 97% thought they should avoid exercise before the sessions, only 60% still believed that after the sessions. The authors concluded that:

> These observations support the hypothesis that the cognitive behavior therapy was effective because of a specific effect on illness perpetuating beliefs and coping behavior.

The authors refer to a collaborative approach to re-evaluating patients' illness beliefs but show no evidence of paying any attention to the patients' illness beliefs; indeed, they seem to triumph in having changed them.

The problem with evaluating the role of CBT in CFS is that it seems to have been applied with a view to providing explanations as to why the person has developed the illness, rather than as an aid to better coping by those who have the illness. The technique has also been applied with some considerable success in physical illnesses other than CFS, such as AIDS and cancer, where no one makes the assumption that psychological feelings are *perpetuating factors*. Nor do they assume a causal relationship in such conditions. (Folkman and Greer, 2000; Greer *et al.*, 1992; Kidman and Edelman, 1999).

The unfortunate implications behind these psychological techniques is that CFS sufferers have caused their own illness by their weakness and negativity. While this negative connotation persists there will be no enthusiasm for the treatment. We have heard it argued that no such causal implications are assumed by this model but have then heard these same practitioners ridiculing and denigrating the patients who resist their models. As Epstein, Quill and McWhinney (1999) have commented:

> All illnesses in all patients have emotional and social considerations … Rather than invoking emotions and social factors in only those illnesses whose solutions remain unexplained, a biopsychosocial approach requires simultaneous exploration of emotions, the social context, and physical markers of disease in all but the most minor illness.

So the problem with modalities such as CBT and graded exercise programs is that they are overdependent on systems, theories and practitioners for their success. Therapist-centered treatment, like doctor-centered treatment, seems only to be successful when the affected person consents to the evaluated therapy. The need for the person to be convinced, against his or her will, of the psychological origins of the *perpetuating factors* in their illness seems unnecessarily demeaning to the person and an odd start for the use of a very valuable therapy. In addition, interpretation of these trials is difficult because there seems to be a suggestion that the power of the therapist is the most important factor in their success. This also constitutes a problem because the RCTs which were successful required 16 hours of therapist time over four months per CFS patient. Most family doctors would judge that an hour's consultation each week with such patients would also make a significant difference to their functioning. Even in conditions such as depression there is dispute over the effectiveness of CBT (Thase et al., 2000) and so this form of treatment cannot be considered a practical solution for the vast majority of sufferers.

Patient self-management

The goals of the patient are largely self-evident: to get rid of the troubling symptoms and return to their pre-illness state. However, this is not a simple task, as previous chapters have outlined. With no simple pill-taking or procedural routine leading to recovery, both physician and patient must set realistic goals for the management of the condition. The patient wants to get on with some sort of life, and this is fraught with difficulties, given the interwoven issues of the physical illness, the social and environmental settings and the lack of a ready biomedical answer. It is made all the more difficult by the reticence of the physician in being drawn into the swamp of concomitant psychosocial circumstances of a particular patient's life. It is often said that doctors just do not have the time, or the expertise, to assist someone in these areas, but our reluctance is more often rooted in our fear of ineffectiveness, uncertainty and conflict. We would rather not risk losing perspective and experiencing a sense of failure. We need to realise that the physician aspects of such relationships must involve such risks, and that blaming or referring the patient when the going gets rough are not the only options open to us. Person-centering demands a partnership in these difficult times and the physician can benefit personally from the reflection and mentorship provided by this 'difficult patient'. Reframing the goals of treatment toward functional improvement, maintaining a therapeutic relationship and avoiding iatrogenic harm may help remoralize the physician and encourage the patient.

Another aspect of the refuge principle is the patient-centered approach in which the doctor and the person with CFS set clear goals and identify their respective roles in achieving those goals. Such methods have been employed within the psychological disciplines but these have not been well received by most CFS patients, largely because of the implications of having to accept blame for the illness. However, there are frameworks for managing the symptomatic and psychosocial issues that go with living 'between office visits'. A good example is the approach employed by Siegel (1990) in groups such as Exceptional Cancer Patients.

An action research project undertaken by one of the authors (Denz-Penhey and Murdoch, 1993; Denz-Penhey et al., 1999) addressed the issues of just what the person who was ill could do to improve their symptom control and their whole quality of life. Its aim was to identify useful and respectful frameworks that could be accepted as self-evident and which would arouse no controversy when recommended. There were several premises. The first was that there were ways of functioning, even when severely ill, which would improve the quality of life. The second was that the people who were ill were the ideal people to identify and formulate the approach and the issues, not professionals coming with an already identified set of assumptions. The author had recovered herself from the illness, as had two of her children, and she had several friends who had also recovered. A key aspect to recovery had been the daily practice of relaxation and/or meditation and this observation was offered to the action research participants. It was found, though, that this, while accepted, was not incorporated into their lifestyle. One of the important assumptions of action research is that the participants are never wrong and so the issues surrounding the observation were explored. Was it that relaxation and meditation did not work, was it disrespectful, or was it that something else had to happen first? The various groups in the project all found that relaxation and meditation made the person who was ill acutely aware of their symptoms and their psychosocial stressors. They also felt blamed for having any such psychosocial problems. This was experienced as intensely unpleasant and they naturally desired not to use the relaxation and meditation that precipitated such feelings. However, it was found that when they shut down their feelings in order to reduce symptom levels, they also stopped identifying those things which they could change and which drained their energy. Initially, it appeared to be a Catch 22 situation.

The first step, then, came to be to identify all the things that the person who was ill was doing that were right. At all costs the sense of blame that was so debilitating had to be avoided, as it prevented a rational self-assessment that was needed prior to making change. This became a 'self-management check-in' (see Box 7.1).

The person who was ill gave themselves a tick for each time they did something right (that is, it contributed to an improved quality of life) and a plus (+) for any time they became aware that the outcome was not useful. What was not allowed was a cross (×) that might indicate blame and hence shut down useful feedback. Self-awareness of the need to change was necessary prior to change occurring.

The second step was for the group to identify needs that were not being met and which contributed to their personal discomfort or which were major energy drainers. After various models were tried Maslow's hierarchy of needs (Maslow, 1987) was modified (see Figure 7.1).

The important change here was that this turned the traditional triangle upside down. When self-actualization was at the top of the pyramid the whole model was found to be irrelevant, but when it was turned up the other way the participants were quickly able to see which needs were not being met. It was quite common for them to admit to not getting sufficient fresh air, keeping themselves warm enough, drinking enough water, eating appropriately, going

> **Box 7.1** *The self-management check-in*
>
> **Physical**: including visits to the doctor, naturopath, etc; meeting sleep and rest needs; deep relaxation, meditation, etc; tai chi, yoga, massage, etc; diet and exercise.
>
> **Self-acceptance and self-esteem**: feelings, self-talk and activities.
>
> **Relationships**: partner, family, work, all social contacts.
>
> **Values and principles**: reflection on and action, particularly in relation to time management, priority and boundary setting. Religious beliefs and faith come in here for those to whom it is important.
>
> **Unfinished business**: becoming aware of, and dealing with, anything from the past that causes stress and gets in the way of the healing process.
>
> **Fun, enjoyment and humour**: exploration of when, where and what worked for them.
>
> **Creativity**: activities that could be considered to be art or craft came under this heading.
>
> **Future and dreams**: looking beyond the immediate, to that which was drawing them forward.

to the toilet regularly or getting enough rest. Very few participants got as much rest as they needed and this is interesting when compared to the warnings from the psychiatric lobby who suggest that people with CFS should be steered away from looking to rest as otherwise they might go to bed indefinitely. The key question in relation to meeting of needs was 'Is a lack contributing to my discomfort or to energy draining from me and if so, what can I do about it?'

The answers to these questions lead to the development of the rest of the self-management plan. In order for needs to be met, participants needed to reflect on their roles, the values and principles on which they based their life, the way they set priorities and managed their time, the boundaries they had to set so that they could have their own needs met, and the short- and long-term consequences ('future checks') of any change they might like to put into effect. The other additional check to be made was that they were in a shared reality with some other respected person. It is difficult enough being ill and making changes in ones life, but becoming a crank because one does not have a shared reality with anyone becomes a much worse problem.

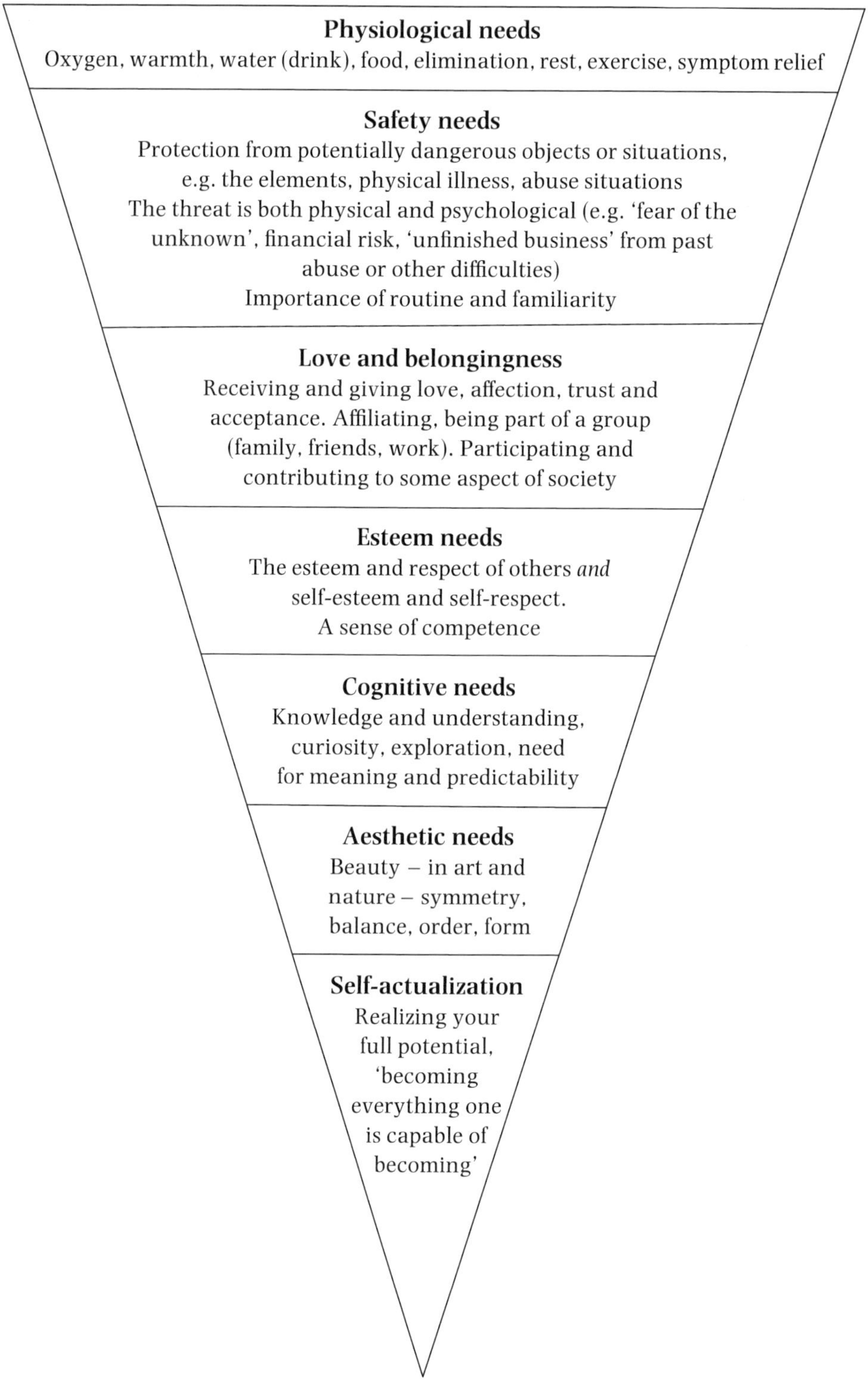

Physiological needs
Oxygen, warmth, water (drink), food, elimination, rest, exercise, symptom relief

Safety needs
Protection from potentially dangerous objects or situations, e.g. the elements, physical illness, abuse situations
The threat is both physical and psychological (e.g. 'fear of the unknown', financial risk, 'unfinished business' from past abuse or other difficulties)
Importance of routine and familiarity

Love and belongingness
Receiving and giving love, affection, trust and acceptance. Affiliating, being part of a group (family, friends, work). Participating and contributing to some aspect of society

Esteem needs
The esteem and respect of others *and* self-esteem and self-respect.
A sense of competence

Cognitive needs
Knowledge and understanding, curiosity, exploration, need for meaning and predictability

Aesthetic needs
Beauty – in art and nature – symmetry, balance, order, form

Self-actualization
Realizing your full potential, 'becoming everything one is capable of becoming'

Figure 7.1 Hierarchy of needs (adapted from Maslow)

Box 7.2 *Self-management action plan*

Be gentle
Accept myself
Who I am, Where I am, How I am, Why I think I am the way I am

Take charge of my life

Make time for reflection on needs, roles,
values and principles,
boundary and priority setting,
time management,
'reality checks', 'future checks'

Do awareness-raising and relaxation exercises

DO WHAT IS IMPORTANT TO ME
moment by moment

Deal with energy drainers,
internal conflict, resistances,
drivenness,
general discomfort

An unexpected key to recovery was discovered after a Christmas break during the study. Two research groups were being undertaken concurrently. After Christmas, one group had a number of participants who had recovered during the break and most of the rest of them had a vast improvement in health. The health status and general profiles on entry were very similar so the recoveries could not be attributed to differences there. Exploration identified that participants' sense of self-acceptance had reached a critical level just prior to the holiday break. This gave them the sense they were able to be in charge of their life and they negotiated time and conditions which allowed them to meet their rest and self-care needs over Christmas. This self-acceptance had largely not occurred for members of the other group. The finding of the importance of self-acceptance in relation to maximizing health outcomes and patient self-care has a direct relevance to the general practitioner. This underlines the need for the doctor to affirm his or her respect for the patient in the course of every consultation. Perhaps what is necessary is to ask ourselves as doctors why it is that our regard for patients is dependent on their diagnosis. Instead, we must learn and respect the patient's story and like a skilled actor we must try to enter the sacred space of the individual we are trying to help. The word *try* is important, for success is never assured and we must remember that the highest accolade to be achieved may be the familiar one often given by decent, honest people.

> Doc, ya done all ya could, and I want you to know we appreciate it. (Loxtercamp, 1991)

Once study participants were able to undertake the first parts of the self-management plan and their self-acceptance had increased, then undertaking the 'awareness-raising and relaxation exercises', as we called the meditation and progressive muscular relaxation, were not perceived as being a problem. The increased awareness of symptoms and psychosocial stressors became a useful feedback mechanism which lead to improved quality of life.

Being ill takes up a lot of time. When the person who was ill started doing the self-management program it also took time, but it was the general consensus that it took no more time than simply being ill. The suggestion was that during some of the hours of required rest, the person could undertake the reflection suggested on the self-management action plan. This did not need to be heavy self-absorption. A gentle self-questioning with useful non-judgemental reflection was generally more helpful.

Once a person started to undertake good self-care it was frequently commented by family and friends that the person had become 'selfish' and would no longer meet all the needs of others. This needs to be seen for what it is: a selfishness on the part of the family and friends who require the ill person to fulfill the needs of others prior to meeting their own needs. They were also seen to be 'giving in' to the symptoms when they appeared to manage before. 'Appeared to manage' are the operative words. Before undertaking the self-management they still had the symptoms. They just did nothing about changing their personal situation to reduce the symptom levels and improve their own quality of life. Others assumed that prior to self-management the person had managed well. Now the ill person acknowledged the symptoms and the need for some change. Family and friends saw this as a backward step. Taking charge of their own care and drawing boundaries around what they were prepared to accept and undertake was perceived as a problem to relationships rather than a personal re-evaluation which would assist in recovery.

It may be of reassurance to significant others that those who have vastly improved their quality of life and those who have recovered could not be perceived to have 'stayed selfish'. Once they were in charge of their lives and the symptom levels had improved, they were able to live by their values and principles which usually included being caring of others.

Continuing care

Of course the patient will continue to visit the doctor for routine care and it is important to realize that, however difficult the course of CFS might be, the person continues at the same risk of other problems and needs help in preventing common health problems in the same way as other patients in the practice. Having CFS does not confer immunity from all the common disorders; indeed, there is some possibility that the risk of cardiovascular or malignant disease may be increased due to cardiac deconditioning or immune deficiency. This is a good reason for continued active involvement of a generalist or family physician.

The setting is the comfortable, trusting consultation and there has to be open discussion on '*What to do if and when . . .*'. Descriptions of the illness given so far have indicated that it is likely to last for a long time and it is wise at the beginning to discuss what is likely to happen and what might be helpful.

We should always be alert in the interpretation of new symptoms and keep an open mind to the diagnostic possibilities. Experience has shown that there can be a delay in the diagnosis of other disorders if symptoms are always assumed to be those of CFS, and at worst these could be life-threatening.

Management of some presenting problems

What are the patient's most pressing symptoms at the present time? Are they part of the CFS or should we look elsewhere for their cause?

Fatigue

Fatigue is a continuing problem and the judicious use of rest is an important discovery for most people. There is usually a choice to be made between competing activities. Total bedrest is probably not a good idea because of the dangers of deconditioning but in some severe cases it cannot be avoided (Sharpe and Wessely, 1998). There are those who make much of placing these extreme problems in the context of Victorian ladies who went to bed permanently. Such accounts seem to amuse inveterate attenders at conferences but are not helpful to the doctors and patients facing real difficulties with severe fatigue. Seldom is the refuge of the hospital bed open to such people and there are many examples of families who have had to cope with no help. Relapsing and less-severe fatigue needs a symptomatic response. They should rest and sleep when required. In the self-management research the groups found it useful to distinguish between sleep, 'blob-out' time (i.e. non-thinking, non-activity), rest and reflection time and rest and reading or television time. All appeared to be needed. The 'blob-out' time was the one most frequently missed and yet needed.

There are those who wish to reduce all exercise to the absolute minimum in order to reduce the amount of sleep and rest required. However, it was found in the self-management groups that the deconditioning was reduced and social functioning improved if patient-chosen activity that improved their quality of life was encouraged. The key to this was that it had to be an activity that would improve their quality of life and functioning. It could not be just to fulfill a family or social demand. Time, then, had to be allowed for the additional rest and sleep needed to recover over the next period of time (hours or days).

Pain and muscle ache

These are a real problem and clinically they can be detected by testing in muscle groups, such as the thenar muscle, for evidence of exquisite tenderness. Often the most effective remedy is aspirin rather than paracetamol, although care has to be taken that the person does not have a sensitivity to the drug. It is also advisable for it to be taken with meals. There is often an overlap between chronic pain syndrome and CFS and a study in Dunedin suggested that CFS was a subpopulation of chronic pain. Where pain is a dominating feature in CFS, it might be useful, rather than persisting with analgesics that do not work, to refer to a pain clinic for advice.

Sleep disturbances

While sleep disorder is very common in CFS people, it should be remembered that up to 22% of the population in European countries were regarded as having severe insomnia. Benzodiazepines have been the pharmacologic agents of choice for the treatment of insomnia, but there is reason to exercise caution with their use; their overall benefit compared with placebo appears to be minor, and they are often associated with adverse cognitive effects, already a feature of CFS. The recent use of melatonin in sleep disorders (Kayumov *et al.*, 2000) has led some to believe that this may be helpful in CFS, particularly since there is some evidence of hypothalamic dysfunction (*see* Chapter 3). However, melatonin has been shown to have normal levels in CFS (Korszun *et al.*, 1999) and the conclusion of the study was that there was no rationale for using it in treatment. However, many people with CFS find that melatonin is their sleeping tablet of choice.

Depression

Many studies have shown that depressive illness is an important co-morbidity in people with CFS. The Dunedin study (Blakely *et al.*, 1991) quoted above, using the Beck Depression Inventory, found that 52% had moderate or severe depression compared to 38% of the chronic pain group and 11% of age and sex matched controls (However, this also means that 48% of those with CFS had no depression). Likewise the prevalence of psychiatric disorder as measured by the General Health Questionnaire (GHQ) or the Structured Clinical Interview for DSM-IV (SCID) has also been high. In the Dunedin study this was 58% whereas the recent Chicago study showed a level of current psychiatric diagnosis of 54.8%. On an individual level, people with CFS can be expected to be vulnerable to bouts of depression and to phobia and panic attacks. Although RCTs of antidepressants have shown no benefit, they can sometimes be beneficial to individuals. Care must be taken to start at a low dose (50%) since people with CFS can be unduly sensitive to such drugs. The rationale of treatment should also be fully explained and a chemical view of depression caused by lack of neurotransmitters can often be much more helpful than the use of language that implies failure and guilt in causing depression. Given the long time that many CFS people have to wait for a rational explanation for their symptoms, it is perhaps surprising that many more do not develop depression, panic disorder and other psychiatric problems.

Bowel symptoms and food sensitivities

There is also considerable overlap between CFS and irritable bowel syndrome (IBS) which is marked by symptoms of abdominal pain and diarrhea without evidence of physical changes in pathology tests. Changes in bowel symptoms in CFS people can be very difficult to handle on the individual patient level because new disorders such as malignant or inflammatory bowel disease can still occur. This emphasizes the point that day to day management in any patient must be done on an individual basis because textbook examples of any diagnosis only occur as models in the minds of researchers and authors, and not in real individuals in the real world. In that world, decisions will have to be made about when to refer to specialist colleagues for endoscopies and biopsies and tests will have to be done to see if other problems exist, such as gluten or lactose intolerance. Such explorations have to be done with the full consent of both patients and doctors and one of the roles of the scientifically trained doctor will be to retain both a healthy scepticism and the regard of the patient. The desired outcome is the relief of the symptom and any experimentation in dietary manipulation should start with a joint decision about when that outcome is going to be measured.

Menstrual and pregnancy issues

About two-thirds of CFS sufferers are women in the child-bearing age and there are many problems surrounding the issues of contraception, menstrual problems, pregnancy, lactation and menopause which are beyond the scope of this book. With regard to symptom control, women with CFS often report that there is a pre-menstrual worsening of their CFS symptoms, and that they are unduly prone to pre-menstrual tension.

No one doctor has met a large number of women who have become pregnant when they had CFS but the general impression is that symptoms tend to improve during the pregnancy. The problems seem to come during labor with the additional exertion required and in the busy time following the birth.

Sharing care with others

When symptoms are slow to disappear as is certainly the case in CFS, there will always be the desire to try new therapies and to seek other opinions as to the cause of the problem. As we have already said, most people with CFS would do literally anything, go anywhere and spend all they could afford if there was even a small chance that they could feel better. Family and community networks are soon aware of the problem faced by one of their number and this is illustrated by our case study where Wendy's parents wish to send her to the States to seek help for the problem.

People are often embarrassed to raise these issues with their regular doctor as they fear that it may be misinterpreted as meaning that they are dissatisfied with the service they have received. If the question as to whether the doctor has heard of this practitioner or treatment is raised, it should be answered honestly and not defensively. Asking the question does not necessarily mean that the person is dissatisfied with the doctor's performance so far. In fact, it probably means that there is a depth of trust in the relationship since most people are reluctant to tell their usual doctor that they are trying other treatments. A defensive response from the doctor is probably expected and so is unlikely to be helpful.

Many doctors have difficulty when confronted with a patient determined to pursue alternative treatments and wonder how much encouragement or discouragement is appropriate, especially in those cases where the beliefs and mythology surrounding the alternative approach is contrary to medical and/ or mainline Western thought.

Rather than providing a list of complementary approaches and a critique of them, we aim to suggest some frameworks within which a doctor might consider them and best advise their patients. Complementary approaches can be subdivided into three main areas: nutritional, physical and emotional/spiritual.

Nutritional

The view of many of those coming from a nutritional perspective is that the body is compromised and is therefore not fully utilizing the digestive system. Even if there is sufficient intake of nutrients they are not being absorbed. The suggestion is that the patient should flood their body with top nutrition. Herbal, vitamin and mineral (often colloidal) supplements are recommended. It is often suggested to use dietary and vitamin supplements for adrenal support and to reduce the work on the liver. Additional vitamins to combat the stress affect of the illness is unlikely to be harmful. Homeopathy would also come under this heading.

Physical

This would include chiropractic, kinesiology, body-balancing to increase energy, gentle manipulation of the muscle and skeletal systems, massage,

Feldenkrais, Touch for Health and Hakomi. Again, none of these approaches is likely to be harmful and may provide the person with some important self-management techniques.

Emotional/spiritual

The theme of a great many working in this area is that the person's body is crying out for nurturing self-care and has become exhausted. At its best, these approaches can assist the patient to deal with heightened supersensitivity to emotions and avoid denigrating, other-oriented demands.

Cautions

It is important to understand that those who practise complementary therapies frequently have the same rigid models of causation that characterize most medical practitioners. In fact, they can be more rigid because there is usually no formal evidence collected as to the overall effectiveness of the therapy. The real problem facing both patients and doctors trying to assess the worth of these therapies is that there is little quality control of practitioners and their disciplines tend to be therapy-centered rather than patient-centered. Some are obviously cranks and in these cases we have a duty to protect the individual from fraud. For example, if a patient with CFS asked her doctor about the validity of a therapist in another country who had asked her to send him a recent photograph from which he was able to diagnose food sensitivities for a fee of $20, a frank answer would have to be forthcoming.

We should encourage the person to keep an open mind as to whether they are getting the results from the complementary approaches they try. The experience of many is that they can pay large amounts of money for very little positive result. However, doctors cannot afford to be too critical as those with CFS pay the medical profession large amounts for very little positive results also. Both patients and doctors should remember that CFS is a multifactorial condition and just as it is unlikely that any one pharmacological intervention is likely to produce a cure, so it is unlikely that one complementary approach will produce a cure. Some patients go seeking the magic pill, potion or therapy that will make all the symptoms go away and try everything serially: 'tried this, didn't work; tried that, didn't work'.

A more useful way to consider using complementary approaches is to encourage the patient to consider how much the approach of choice improves their quality of life and whether they consider the practitioner is respectful of them and their condition. This is especially important when the beliefs and mythology that underpin the approach are not part of the patient's normal community reality. It is difficult enough for a person to deal with the multitude of symptoms at the best of times and most would want to avoid being considered a crank by friends and family. However, there are many cases where emotional support has been respectful and physical improvement has occurred as a result of dealing with such complementary health practitioners.

Clinical experience has suggested two additional areas of caution. There are some complementary practitioners who recommend drastic changes in diet such as a complete restriction of protein. This is very unwise and can leave the patient further compromised. Rotation diets and diets that exclude whole families of food is also a frequent recommendation. This can be severely socially debilitating and we have found it seldom to be more than a very short-term solution for a reduction in symptoms as they become sensitive to more and more of the food groups over a period of time. We have found it more useful to focus on widening life options rather than reducing them. Hence we encourage active self-management of symptoms rather than attempting to identify individual foods or food groups that might be contributing to the symptoms. As the health improves with good self-management, then the food sensitivities reduce.

Massage has been reported to be very helpful by many, but some practitioners use massage that is too harsh for people with CFS. The patient's experience should be the guide: it should enhance their sense of well-being and quality of life.

What do we do when it's not working?

We need to be aware of the fact that there is a percentage of people who do not recover from CFS. Because we do not know what causes CFS it is very difficult to identify why this should be. Those who continue downhill into a lifestyle of total invalidism and apparent helplessness often suffer needlessly because it is often assumed, by orthodox and complementary health professionals, that they 'enjoy' poor health and use their symptoms to manipulate their environment.

> Roseanne (in her 40s) became very unwell with a flu virus shortly after being divorced from her husband of 25 years. She was left to look after three of the six children still at home. For several years she had been virtually bedridden and she had lost all confidence in doctors or healers of any kind. Having regained some mobility and self-respect, she asked if she could attend the family physician (JCM) from time to time, on the strict understanding that he would prescribe no drugs but would provide information and preventive advice.

In our communities there are people who are totally isolated from healthcare providers but who have courageously endured long years of chronic illness.

'Hanging on in there' is very important for these people and their families, and if physicians are asked to assist with their care it is important that we do not scare them off by putting too many conditions on our involvement. Often we may be the only link they have with medical care and the alternative to our involvement is no medical contact at all. To put it simply, we have to stay patient-centered, give unconditional positive regard, encourage good self-management by the patient and their families and give symptomatic care when possible. Continuity of respectful care has, on occasions, to be sufficient in itself. We also have to resist the temptation to feel guilty about our lack of success. Much as we would like all to recover, sometimes that does not occur.

Conclusion

From what we have learned about CFS in this book, it is obvious that treatment has got to be used in its broadest sense when applied to this syndrome. The studies of treatment do seem to suggest that people with CFS are willing to comply with treatment regimes but that there has been a disappointing response where one treatment has been compared to placebo. The treatments which have shown promise are those such as exercise programs, cognitive behavioral therapy and self-management programs, all of which have many possible reasons for their success.

The lessons of immediate care may once again be applied to our approach to treatment in CFS. In the real world, when we are confronted with a collapse we deal with it on an individual level, using evidence-based treatments if these are available. If they are not available, or if they do not work in that individual, we don't just stand there, we do something, using a number of strategies which experience and training has taught us to be useful in resuscitation. Some, such as external cardiac massage and mouth-to-mouth resuscitation we do always. Others, such as the use of DC shock or certain injections, we use if they are clinically indicated. At the end of the day, we judge our success on the survival of the patient and our own feelings about whether we performed satisfactorily. Standing idly by and declaring that we have no evidence that anything will work is not acceptable, neither is declaring that we are not expert enough to carry out the procedures.

The same general principles apply when a person with CFS consults the doctor. Delay in diagnosis is the usual problem and reluctance to classify people as CFS is the major issue in most cases. We should not hesitate to offer a refuge; we do not fear dependence as an outcome in treating cardiogenic shock. The equivalent of external cardiac massage and mouth-to-mouth resuscitation and oxygen is the assurance to the person that we understand their problem and that we will be there for them as long as we are needed. This should include discussion about the likely course of the illness, with added optimism being present the younger the person is. Experience teaches that most people are very much better once they have had this therapy.

Short-term treatment strategies are important to reassure the person affected that their doctor has some knowledge of the condition and how to treat it. These could include such treatments as a short course of low-dose steroids, antidepressants or vitamin B12 injections. It is important that we give these on the basis that they have helped some people but by no means all.

The timeframe of the CFS emergency is of course different from that of immediate care. Resuscitation should take place immediately and diagnosis should be complete within a month. A further three months of short-term strategies is then feasible, with a mutual assessment at monthly intervals of how things are going with regard to major problems and symptom control.

In the longer term it may be important to give some thought to the organization of small groups where we can talk about self-management or exercise programs as a possible option. The use of the self-management approach as a basis for these groups is a possibility. There are other people such as counselors and support group co-ordinators who may be appropriate to involve. What is very important is to have a plan.

All of this seems very trivial, even humdrum, in the light of the sophisticated research which has been published, but for Wendy Jones, it would have been a life-saver. The treatment which Dr Rose arranged for her created a world in which she was alone, where her husband and relatives were unsupportive, where the social services refused to support her and where her children and husband were put at risk. While there is no guarantee that this treatment regime will alleviate her symptoms, she will leave the person-centered consultation with a clear feeling of support and knowledge, with a believable story to tell her family, with a certificate qualifying her for social support. She will return to a different world; not an ideal world but a better world.

It will be better because she has helped to design it. In Dr Rose she found a rigid practitioner who could only solve problems by the routine application of facts, rules and procedures derived from a fixed body of professional knowledge. Each time she saw him, she knew she was going nowhere and she left his office with a solution which did not fit her circumstances. Hopefully in Dr Lane she has found someone who engages in *professional artistry* (Schon, 1990). In the words of Schon this is someone who, faced with an unfamiliar situation where there is no obvious fit between the characteristics of the situation and the available body of theories and techniques, will make design adjustments and by *reflection-in-action*, help to design a world in which Wendy and the family can survive the horrors and the rigors of a nasty illness. In time she may get better. She may not, but at least she will be able to live within the resources which she has.

References

Behan PO, Behan WMH and Horrobin D (1990) Effect of high doses of essential fatty acids on the post-viral fatigue syndrome. *Acta Neurol Scand.* **82**: 209–16.

Berger J (1967) *A Fortunate Man: the story of a country doctor.* The Penguin Press, London, UK.

Blakely AA, Howard R, Sosich R et al. (1991) Psychiatric symptoms, personality and ways of coping in chronic fatigue syndrome. *Psychol. Med.* **21**: 347–62.

Cleare AJ, Heap E, Malhi GS et al. (1999) Low-dose hydrocortisone in chronic fatigue syndrome: a randomised cross-over trial. *Lancet.* **353**: 455–8.

Cochrane AL and Moore F (1971) Expected and observed values for the prescription of vitamin B12 in England and Wales. *Br J Prev Soc Med.* **25**: 147–51.

Cox IM, Campbell MJ and Dowson D (1991) Red cell magnesium and chronic fatigue syndrome. *Lancet.* **337**: 757–60.

Deale A, Chalder T, Marks I and Wessely S (1997) Cognitive behavior therapy for chronic fatigue syndrome: a randomized controlled trial. *Am J Psychiatry.* **154**: 408–14.

Denz-Penhey H and Murdoch JC (1993) General practitioners acceptance of the validity of chronic fatigue syndrome as a diagnosis. *N Z Med J.* **106**: 122–4.

Denz-Penhey H, Tilyard M, Shaw R, Harvey R (1999) Patient self-management in chronic fatigue syndrome: an action research study. *N Z Fam Physician.* **26**(1): 43–50.

Egan E (1985) *Such a Vision of the Street: Mother Teresa – the spirit and the work.* Sidgwick & Jackson, London, UK.

Ellis FR and Nasser S (1973) A pilot study of vitamin B12 in the treatment of tiredness. *Br J Nutr.* **30**(2): 277–83.

Epstein RM, Quill, TE and McWhinney IR (1999) Somatization reconsidered: incorporating the patient's experience of illness. *Arch Intern Med.* **159**: 215–22.

Folkman S and Greer S (2000) Promoting psychological well-being in the face of serious illness: when theory, research and practice inform each other. *Psychooncology.* **9**: 11–19.

Forsyth LM, Preuss HG, McDowell AL et al. (1999) Therapeutic effects of oral NADH on the symptoms of patients with chronic fatigue syndrome. *Ann Allergy Asthma Immunol.* **82**: 185–91.

Fox M (1979) *A Spirituality Named Compassion.* Harper & Row, San Francisco, CA.

Fulcher KY and White PD (1997) Randomised controlled trial of graded exercise in patients with chronic fatigue syndrome. *BMJ.* **314**: 1647–52.

Greer S, Moorey S, Baruch J et al. (1992) Adjuvant psychological therapy for patients with cancer: a prospective randomised trial. *BMJ.* **304**: 675–80.

Guyatt G, Sackett D, Taylor DW et al. (1986) Determining optimal therapy-randomised trials in individual patients. *NEJM.* **314**: 889–92.

Kaslow JE, Rucker L and Onishi R (1989) Liver extract–folic acid–cyanocobalamin vs placebo for chronic fatigue syndrome. *Arch Intern Med.* **149**: 2501–3.

Kayumov L, Zhdanova IV, Shapiro CM (2000) Melatonin, sleep, and circadian rhythm disorders. *Semin Clin Neuropsychiatry.* **5**: 44–55.

Kidman A and Edelman S (1999) *Taking Charge. Strategies for managing the psychological aspects of cancer.* Psych-Oncology Research Unit, University of Technology, Sydney, Australia.

Kieburtz KD, Giang DW, Schiffer RB and Vakil N (1991) Abnormal vitamin B12 metabolism in human immunodeficiency virus infection. *Arch Neurol.* **48**: 312–14.

Korszun A, Sackett-Lundeen L, Papadopoulos E *et al.* (1999) Melatonin levels in women with fibromyalgia and chronic fatigue syndrome. *J Rheumatol.* **26**: 2675–80.

Lindebaum J, Healton EB, Savage DG *et al.* (1988) Neuropsychiatric disorders caused by cobalamin deficiency in the absence of anemia or macrocytosis. *NEJM.* **318**: 1720–8.

Lloyd AR, Hickie I, Wakefield D, Boughton C and Dwyer J (1990) A double-blind, placebo-controlled trial of intravenous immunoglobulin therapy in patients with chronic fatigue syndrome. *Am J Med.* **89**: 561–8.

Lloyd A, Hickie I, Brockman A *et al.* (1993) Immunologic and psychological therapy for patients with chronic fatigue syndrome. *Am J Med.* **94**: 197–203.

Loxtercamp D (1991) Being there: on the place of the family physician. *J Am Board Fam Pract.* **4**: 354–60.

Maslow AH (1987) *A Theory of Human Motivation.* Harper & Row, New York.

McKenzie R, O'Fallon A, Dale J *et al.* (1998) Low-dose hydrocortisone for treatment of chronic fatigue syndrome: a randomized controlled trial. *JAMA.* **280**: 1061–6.

Natelson BH, Cheu J, Pareja J *et al.* (1996) Randomized, double-blind, controlled placebo-phase–in trial of low-dose phenelzine in the chronic fatigue syndrome. *Psychopharmacol (Berl).* **124**: 226–30.

Peterson PK, Shepard J, Macres M *et al.* (1990) A controlled trial of intravenous immunoglobulin-G in chronic fatigue syndrome. *Am J Med.* **89**: 554–60.

Peterson PK, Pheley A, Schroeppel J *et al.* (1998) A preliminary placebo-controlled cross-over trial of fludrocortisone for chronic fatigue syndrome. *Arch Intern Med.* **158**: 908–14.

Plioplys AV and Plioplys S (1997) Amantadine and L-carnitine treatment of chronic fatigue syndrome. *Neuropsychobiol.* **35**: 16–23.

Reid S, Chalder T, Cleare A, Hotopf M and Wessely S (2000) Chronic fatigue syndrome. Extracts from 'Clinical Evidence'. *BMJ.* **320**: 292–6.

Rowe KS (1997) Double-blind randomized controlled trial to assess the efficacy of intravenous immunoglobulin for the management of chronic fatigue syndrome in adolescents. *J Psychiatric Res.* **31**: 133–47.

Schon DA (1990) *Educating the Reflective Practitioner.* Jossey-Bass Publishers, San Francisco, CA.

See DM and Tilles JG (1996) Alpha-interferon treatment of patients with chronic fatigue syndrome. *Immunol Invest.* **25**: 153–64.

Sharpe M and Wessely S (1998) Putting the rest cure to rest – again. *BMJ.* **316**: 796.

Sharpe M, Hawton K, Simkin S et al. (1996) Cognitive behavioural therapy for the chronic fatigue syndrome: a randomised controlled trial. *BMJ.* **312**: 22–6.

Siegel BS (1990) *Peace, Love and Healing: bodymind communication and the path to self-healing: an exploration.* Harper Perennial Library, New York.

Stott NCH (1983) *Primary Health Care: bridging the gap between theory and practice.* Springer-Verlag, Berlin, Germany.

Straus SE, Dale JK, Tobi M et al. (1988) Acyclovir treatment of the chronic fatigue syndrome: lack of efficacy in a placebo-controlled trial. *NEJM.* **319**: 1692–8.

Strayer DR, Carter WA, Brodsky I et al. (1994) A controlled clinical trial with a specifically configured RNA drug, poly(I) (poly(C12U)), in chronic fatigue syndrome. *Clin Infect Dis.* **Suppl 1**: S88–S95.

Thase ME, Friedman ES, Berman SR et al. (2000) Is cognitive behavior therapy just a 'nonspecific intervention for depression?: a retrospective comparison of consecutive cohorts treated with cognitive behavior therapy or supportive counseling and pill placebo. *J Affect Disord.* **57**: 63–71.

Vercoulen JH, Swanink CM, Zitman FG et al. (1996) Randomised, double-blind, placebo-controlled study of fluoxetine in chronic fatigue syndrome. *Lancet.* **347**: 858–61.

Vollmer-Conna U, Hickie I, Hadzi-Pavlovic D et al. (1997) Intravenous immunoglobulin is ineffective in the treatment of patients with chronic fatigue syndrome. *Am J Med.* **103**: 38–43.

Warren G, McKendrick M and Peet M (1999) The role of essential fatty acids in chronic fatigue syndrome. *Acta Neurol Scand.* **99**: 112–16.

Weardon AJ, Morriss RK, Mullis R et al. (1998) Randomised, double-blind, placebo-controlled treatment trial of fluoxetine and graded exercise for chronic fatigue syndrome. *Br J Psychiatry.* **172**: 485–90.

Index

5-hydroxytryptamine (5HT) 64

aches, muscle 154
acknowledging the condition 123–4
Acquired Immune Deficiency Syndrome (AIDS) 111
active positive/negative, coping strategy 87–9
acyclovir, treatment 144
adolescents 91–3
Advanced Trauma Life Support (ATLS) 8–10
AIDS *see* Acquired Immune Deficiency Syndrome
alcohol abuse 12
amantidine, treatment 143–4
Ampligen, treatment 144
antidepressants, treatment 143
antiviral drugs, treatment 144
approaches
   doctor-centered 5–10, 47–50, 104–6, 122
   emotional treatment 158
   holistic 77–97
   person-centered 10–13
   physical treatment 157–8
   psychological 38–40
   spiritual treatment 158
athletes, overtrained 64
ATLS *see* Advanced Trauma Life Support

behaviors
   CBT 142, 145–7
   improving health 125–6
   manipulative 108–9
belief issues 47–50
Berger, John 15
bowel symptoms, management 156

C-reactive protein 90
cancer 12
care
   continuing 153
   sharing 156–9
carnitine, treatment 143–4
cautions, treatment 158–9
Cawley, Robert 130–2
CBT *see* cognitive behavioral therapy
Center for Communicable Disease, CFS definition 11–12
CFIDS *see* chronic fatigue and immunodeficiency syndrome
children 89–91
chronic fatigue and immunodeficiency syndrome (CFIDS) 15, 62–3
chronic fatigue syndrome (CFS)
   defined 11–13
   describing accurately 19–21
   evolution of criteria 11–13
   cf. fatigue 2
   magnitude of problem 1–25
   natural history 21–2
chronic illness with label, CFS stage 85
chronic illness with no label, CFS stage 83–5
clinical features 54
clinical records, retrospective analysis 3–4
clinician–patient relationship 115–35
cognitive behavioral therapy (CBT) 142, 145–7
community-based problem 58
community, problems with 102–4
compassion 140
complementary therapies 156–9
consultations
   language of 41–2
   person-centered experience 120–2
   phases 10–11

consultations (*continued*)
  times 5
  types 1–2
control
  achieving sense of 131–2
  symptoms 124–5
coping strategies 87–9
corticosteroids, treatment 143
course of illness 79–80
Coxsackie virus 60–2
crash, CFS stage 9–10, 80–2, 101
criteria, CFS 11–13, 19–21
Crohn's disease 89–90

depression, management 155
diabetes 28–9
diagnosis 28–31
  belief issues 47–50
  doctor-centered approach 5–10, 47–50
  getting 35
  patients' views 120, 148–53
  person-centered approach 10–13
  personal experience and 28–33
  psychological 106–7
  shortcuts 29–31
  use/misuse 106–8
Diagnostic and Statistical Manual of Mental Disorders 67–8
diagnostic search for cause, consultation phase 10–11
dietary supplements, treatment 143
disparities, stories 33–40
doctor-centered approach 5–10, 47–50, 104–6, 122
doctor–patient relationship 115–35
doctors
  'being there' 118–22
  patients managing 37
  whole person matching 127–31
documenting testimony 28
Down's syndrome 70, 116, 124
drama, consultation type 1–2, 116

efamol, treatment 143
electroconvulsive therapy 130
emotional treatment approaches 158
endocrine system links 63–5
energy-providing substances, treatment 143–4

Epstein-Barr virus 12, 53, 60–2, 90, 94–5
ESR 90
evaluation 13–14
evidence-based medicine
  testimony 2–4
  see also randomized controlled trials
exclusion criteria 13
exercise programs, treatment 142
experiences
  first 34–5
  illness 27–45, 120–2
  personal, and diagnosis 28–33
explanations, acceptable 122–6

failure, treatments 159–60
family, problems with 102–4
fatigue
  cf. CFS 2
  defined 101
  management 154
first experiences 34–5
flu 80–1
  Tapanui flu 4
food sensitivities
  management 154
  see also nutritional issues
forgetfulness 65, 102–3
Frame, Janet 129–32
functional somatic syndrome 65–6, 106–7
future, research 69–70

General Health Questionnaire (GHQ-12); 67, 107
glandular fever 12, 34–5

headache study 71–2
health behaviors, improving 125–6
hearing, cf. listening 42–3
heartsink patients 42, 84, 122
hepatitis B/C 12
heritage, medicine's positive 28–31
herpes virus 60–2
HIV *see* human immunodeficiency virus
holistic approach 77–97
hormone system links 63–5
human immunodeficiency virus (HIV) 60–2

hyperactivity 42–3
hypothalamo-pituitary-end organ function 63–5

IBS *see* irritable bowel syndrome
idiopathic chronic fatigue 15, 23, 141
illness experience 27–45
  dimensions 120–2
illness model 123
immune dysfunction 62–3
immunoregulatory drugs, treatment 144
influenza *see* flu
irritable bowel syndrome (IBS), management 156

knowledge, four fields 31–3

L-carnitine, treatment 143–4
labelling the illness 39–40, 83–5, 110
  see also naming the illness
laboratory investigations 14
language, of consultations 41–2
lifecycle stages 89–95
  adolescents 91–3
  children 89–91
  mothers 93–4
  older persons 94–5
  pregnancy 93–4
  workforce 94
listening, cf. hearing 42–3
literature, early 54–8
lobby groups 109

Mackenzie criteria 12–13
magnesium, treatment 143
magnitude of problem 1–25
manipulative behavior 108–9
Maslow's needs hierarchy 150
mass hysteria 55–7
mastery, achieving sense of 131–2
matching models, need for 42–4
ME *see* myalgic encephalomyelitis
mechanism model, CFS 71–2
media, war by 108–11
medical records, retrospective analysis 3–4
medical system, problems with 104–6
medicine and science 50–2

medicine's oral tradition 40–2
medicine's positive heritage 28–31
memory, short-term 65, 102–3
menstrual issues, management 156
models
  illness 123
  need for matching 42–4
mothers 93–4
Multitest (CMIM) 63
muscle ache, management 153
myalgic encephalomyelitis (ME) 15, 34–5, 47

NADH *see* nicotinamide adenine dinucleotide
naming and explanation, consultation phase 11
naming the illness 14–15, 140–1
  see also labelling the illness
narcolepsy 12
needs hierarchy, Maslow's 150
neuroimaging studies 64
neurotransmitters 64
nicotinamide adenine dinucleotide (NADH) 143–4
no recovery, CFS stage 86–7
nutritional issues 157
  dietary supplements 143
  food sensitivities 156

obesity 12
older persons 94–5
oral tradition, medicine's 40–2
Oxford Criteria 13

pain, management 154
passive positive/negative, coping strategy 87–9
pathophysiology, search for 47–8
patient–clinician relationship 115–35
patients
  diagnosis views 120, 148–53
  heartsink 42, 84, 122
  managing doctors 37
  self-management 147–53
  whole person matching 127–31
Paul Bunnel test 90
perpetuating factors 146–7
person-centered approach 10–13

person-centered research   58–69
personal experience, diagnosis and
    28–33
physical treatment approaches   157–8
physician–patient relationship   115–35
poliomyelitis   54–5
post-viral fatigue syndrome   36
power, professional   48–50
pregnancy   93–4, 156
prevalence, CFS   16–19, 79, 107
professional power   48–50
prolonged fatigue   15, 16, 19
psychiatric illness   12
psychiatric stigma   39–40
psychological approach   38–40
psychological diagnosis   106–7
psychological impairment   65–9
psychological stigma   39–40

randomized controlled trials (RCTs)
    141–2, 145
recognition of suffering, consultation
    phase   10
records, clinical, retrospective analysis
    3–4
recovery with relapse, CFS stage   85–6
refuge provision   139–40
relapse   85–6
    prevention   126
relationship, patient-clinician   115–35
research   52–72
    directions   70–2
    future development   69–70
retrospective analysis, clinical records
    3–4
ritual, consultation type   2, 116
routine, consultation type   2, 116

Sassall, John   128–9
schools   91
science and medicine   50–2
scientific research, conclusions   145–7
scientifically validated treatments   141–4
screening   14
self-management, patients   147–53
Self-Management Research   35–40
sharing care   156–9
side effects, medication   12

similarities, stories   33–40
sleep disturbances, management   155
societal context   99–114
societal messages   37–8
somatization   50, 107–8
    see also functional somatic syndrome
somatized mental disorder   107–8
sore throat   11, 12, 34–5
spiritual treatment approaches   158
stages
    of illness   80–9
    lifecycle   89–95
stigma, psychological/psychiatric
    label   39–40
stories, CFS   33–40, 122
substance abuse   12
suicide   92–3
symptoms
    control   124–5
    coping with   36–7
    management   153–6

Tapanui flu   4
technical rationality   126
testimony
    documenting   28
    evidence-based medicine   2–4
    patient–clinician relationship
        115–17
thyroid, underactive   12
treatment, finding appropriate   137–64
    antidepressants   143
    antiviral drugs   144
    CBT   142, 145–7
    conclusions   160–1
    conclusions, scientific research
        145–7
    continuing care   153
    corticosteroids   143
    dietary supplements   143
    energy-providing substances   143–4
    exercise programs   142
    failure, treatments   159–60
    immunoregulatory drugs   144
    management, presenting problems
        153–6
    patient self-management   147–53
    RCTs   141–2, 145
    refuge provision   139–40

scientifically validated treatments 141–4
vitamin B12 144

viral cause, continuing search for 60–2
viral illnesses 80–1
  Coxsackie virus 60–2
  Epstein-Barr virus 12, 53, 60–2, 90, 94–5
  herpes virus 60–2
  HIV 60–2
vitamin B12, treatment 144

whole person, understanding the 77–97, 127–31
workforce 94